Palliative Care:
An Oxford Core Text

Christina Faull

Consultant in Palliative Medicine
University Hospital
Birmingham

and

Richard Woof

Clinical lecturer
University of Birmingham

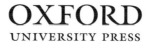

OXFORD
UNIVERSITY PRESS

OXFORD

UNIVERSITY PRESS

Great Clarendon Street, Oxford OX2 6DP

Oxford University Press is a department of the University of Oxford.
It furthers the University's objective of excellence in research, scholarship,
and education by publishing worldwide in

Oxford New York

Auckland Bangkok Buenos Aires Cape Town Chennai
Dar es Salaam Delhi Hong Kong Istanbul Karachi Kolkata
Kuala Lumpur Madrid Melbourne Mexico City Mumbai Nairobi
São Paulo Shanghai Taipei Tokyo Toronto

Oxford is a registered trade mark of Oxford University Press
in the UK and in certain other countries

Published in the United States
by Oxford University Press Inc., New York

©Oxford University Press, 2002

The moral rights of the author have been asserted

Database right Oxford University Press (maker)

First published 2002

All rights reserved. No part of this publication may be reproduced,
stored in a retrieval system, or transmitted, in any form or by any means,
without the prior permission in writing of Oxford University Press,
or as expressly permitted by law, or under terms agreed with the appropriate
reprographics rights organization. Enquiries concerning reproduction
outside the scope of the above should be sent to the Rights Department,
Oxford University Press, at the address above

You must not circulate this book in any other binding or cover
and you must impose this same condition on any acquirer

A catalogue record for this title is
available from the British Library

Library of Congress Cataloguing in Publication Data
(Data available)
ISBN 0 19 263280 9 (Pbk.)

10 9 8 7 6 5 4 3 2

Typeset by EXPO Holdings, Malaysia
Printed on acid-free paper in China

R726.8
.F38
2002

049352119

OXFORD MEDICAL PUBLICATIONS

Palliative Care

Whilst every effort has been made to ensure that the contents of this book are as complete, accurate and up-to-date as possible at the date of writing, Oxford University Press is not able to give any guarantee or assurance that this is the case. Readers are urged to take appropriately qualified medical advice in all cases. The information in this book is intended to be useful to the general reader, but should not be used as a means of self-diagnosis or for the prescription of medication.

Be careful, then, and be gentle about death.
For it is hard to die, it is difficult to go through
the door, even when it opens.

DH Lawrence *All Souls' Day*

Preface

All doctors need to know how best to care for patients with advanced, life limiting disease and those who are dying. Our patients need us to be knowledgeable, skilful and understanding. This book outlines the fundamental principles and facts which will enable you to make a very real difference to our patients and their families. In addition it has been found that by increasing our confidence in providing such care we gain greater professional satisfaction.

The care of patients with advanced and terminal illness can be extremely rewarding but often causes junior and indeed senior clinicians, a considerable amount of discomfort. This is especially so when they feel under confident in their abilities to provide a high quality of symptom management and relief from distress and to communicate appropriately with patients. Patients with advanced disease present some of the most challenging ethical, physical, psychological and social issues to clinicians and indeed to society. Their care requires a true integration of the art and science of medicine. The last part of life is filled with loss, celebration, re-evaluation, regrets, love, suffering, resolution, turmoil and peace. It is small wonder that their care is sometimes uncomfortable!

Palliative care is a fast growing speciality. The success of the hospice movement has resulted in the adoption of palliative care methods into a wide spectrum of health care and they are seen as effective and central to routine clinical practice, both in hospital and the community.

For doctors in training, the General Medical Council has recommended the following:

- Competency in the amelioration of suffering, the relief of pain and the care of the dying person.
- Skills in communication and clinical assessment.
- Development of attitudes which enables doctors to work with people with incurable illness who are facing the certainty of death within their own psycho-social and cultural context.

This book aims to be both a practical resource and to provoke contemplative professional development. Whilst aimed primarily at medical undergraduates and junior doctors, it will be of use to students in other clinical disciplines.

The importance of the palliative care approach to patients is reflected in it being increasingly taught and examined in medical school. As learners you will also have many valuable experiences outside of formal teaching in this area, where palliative care can both assist your clinical practice and satisfy examiners. We know that we all learn in different ways. Some are very good at reading text and remembering, others prefer to learn more by experience. This book aims to appeal to a broad range of learning styles by presenting information in different ways. Hopefully the variety will make it interesting and enjoyable, therefore enhancing your learning.

To make sure the content of the book is appropriate we have used the nationally agreed curriculum on palliative care for undergraduates. This curriculum has been devised by those in the field who assist junior doctors in their work and is used by many lecturers when planning teaching. This means that wherever you are studying or working, you know we have included all the important information. Knowing what you need to know is important for the busy student; you want to be efficient in your learning. To help you we have included this curriculum in questionnaire form so that you can assess your own strengths and weaknesses.

We hope you enjoy this book and by the end feel better prepared to help patients and families at a time of great need.

"Doctors who otherwise pride themselves on careful diagnosis followed by rational and precise treatment so often sink into a mire of mythology and emotions when faced with a dying patient ... Patients are ignored when they most need attention, deceived when they most need someone with the courage to face the predicament with them and, worst of all, left in pain because the doctor fears to use the analgesics readily available to him" Lamerton R 1973 *Care of the Dying*. Priory Press

C. F. and R. W.
March 2002

Dedications

To our children Leo, William and Rory.

Acknowledgements

This book could not have been completed without the support of our partners Alison and Andrew and their generosity in creating the time for us to write. We should also like to thank Catherine Barnes from Oxford University Press for her enthusiasm and professional guidance and Michael Cole for his artistic input.

Cover
A water-colour entitled *The healing touch* reproduced by kind permission of the artist Michele Angelo Petrone. Michele paints and writes of his experience during the treatment of Hodkin's disease.

Cartoon 3 of Chapter 1
A water-colour entitled *The journey to where?* reproduced with kind permission of the artist Michele Angelo Petrone.

Cartoon 4 of Chapter 1
A water-colour entitled *The pain of it all* reproduced with kind permission of the artist Michele Angelo Petrone.

Contents

CHAPTER 1

Introduction. What is palliative care all about? *1*

CHAPTER 2

Taking a palliative care history and handling difficult situations *13*

CHAPTER 3

Psychosocial aspects of palliative care, and why they matter *27*

CHAPTER 4

Decisions around the end of life *43*

CHAPTER 5

Physical symptom control: how to do it well *61*

CHAPTER 6

The syringe driver: a useful way to deliver drugs *87*

CHAPTER 7

Regulations and statutory duties: some rules *101*

CHAPTER 8

Further information about palliative care and useful resources *113*

References *123*

Further reading *125*

Appendix 1
How much palliative medicine do *you* need to learn? *127*

Appendix 2
Drugs you will use frequently for symptom management *137*

Index *139*

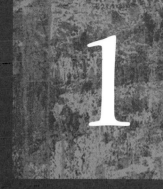

1

CHAPTER 1

Introduction: What is palliative care all about?

♦ What is palliative care? *3*

♦ A little bit of history: some of the key players *7*

♦ Epidemiology for the houseman *8*

♦ How to care well for the dying *9*

♦ Case history exercise: some thoughts on Mrs Jones *11*

CHAPTER 1

Introduction: What is palliative care all about?

I speak of the Prolongation and Utilization of Life, and the Alleviation of Suffering. These may seem subordinate at first, but often they are far from being so in the estimation of the patient. To many life never seems more precious than when they are on the point of losing it; and more gratitude is often testified to the physician when he succeeds in achieving the minor triumph of prolonging life and relieving pain, than in the case where he may have accomplished a perfect restoration to health and ease.

Dr C. J. B. Williams, consulting physician to the Brompton Hospital, First Lumleian lecture to the Royal College of Physicians on *The success and failures of medicine*, 1862.

On my very first day as a medical house officer I was faced with the care of a 56-year-old man, waking up from a temazepam overdose which he had taken because of his incurable lung cancer. He was deeply regretful, both for the hurt he had caused his family and the fact that he had failed to kill himself. He was withdrawn and chose to lie in bed with his eyes tightly closed. I, like many newly qualified doctors, felt ill-equipped to help this man and his family. I muddled through. I remember it as scary. One of those patients I'll never forget. This man and the problems he had didn't fit into the model I had of medicine. Taking his 'history' revealed the physical symptoms of the lung cancer. It all appeared miserable. I felt helpless and struggled with my agreement with his reasons for wanting to die. I wanted to do something to make things better but I couldn't do anything about the cancer.

As a junior doctor you will often be caring for people with incurable fatal conditions, managing the problems of advanced diseases, looking after patients who are dying, and supporting their families. For most new doctors this presents a challenge unlike any other.

None of us wants to 'muddle through' and fail to help patients when they need help most. The speciality of palliative medicine has developed to guide us. Like any other medical discipline there is an evidence base, recommended standards of good practice and a defined curriculum for medical students (Appendix 1). Whatever branch of medicine you eventually specialize in, you will be responsible for patients with palliative care needs and you will need to be confident that you can palliate their symptoms and reduce their distress.

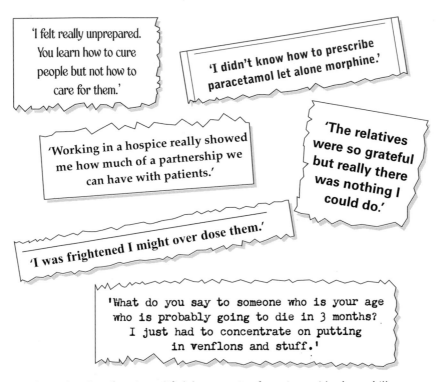

'I felt really unprepared. You learn how to cure people but not how to care for them.'

'I didn't know how to prescribe paracetamol let alone morphine.'

'Working in a hospice really showed me how much of a partnership we can have with patients.'

'The relatives were so grateful but really there was nothing I could do.'

'I was frightened I might over dose them.'

'What do you say to someone who is your age who is probably going to die in 3 months? I just had to concentrate on putting in venflons and stuff.'

1.1 Some thoughts of newly qualified doctors caring for patients with advanced illness

Just because you can't cure them, doesn't mean you can't have a dramatic effect on their quality of life and the way they die. There is *always* something you can do. Palliative care should not be seen as an optional extra, for the patient or for you. It should be an integrated part of the way we all work as doctors.

You have the potential to really make a difference for patients. You can use your knowledge of drugs to alleviate suffering. You can speak with patients to understand what they want and help them get it. As a doctor, you really do have a great chance to help, usually much more than you think.

What is palliative care?

To help us understand how we can best help dying patients, the World Health Organization has agreed a definition and principles of palliative care[1] (see boxes).

What are we aiming for?

The goals of palliative care are to achieve the best possible quality of life for patients and their families, to facilitate adjustment to the many losses they will

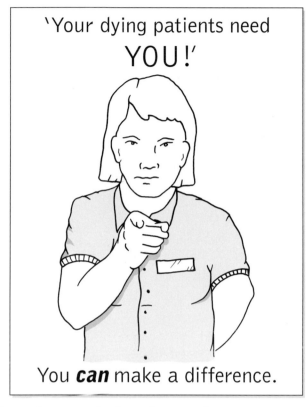

1.2 Palliative care is not an optional extra for your patients

Palliative care

♦ Affirms life and regards dying as a normal process.

♦ Neither hastens nor postpones death.

♦ Provides relief from pain and other distressing symptoms.

♦ Integrates the psychological, physical, social, and spiritual aspects of a patient's care (holism).

♦ Offers a support system to help patients to live as actively as possible until death.

♦ Offers a support system to help the family cope during the patient's illness and in their own bereavement

> *Palliative care* is the active, total (holistic) care of patients and their families by a multiprofessional team when the patient's disease is no longer responsive to curative treatment.

face, and to attain a dignified death with minimum distress in the patient's place of choice.

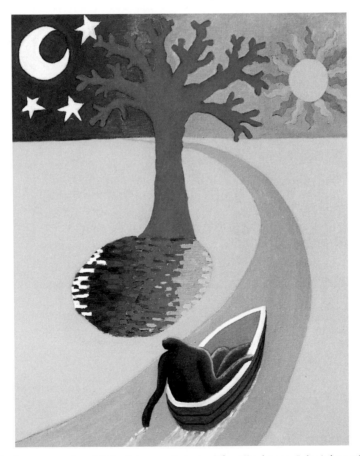

1.3 The journey to where? 'I don't know where my life will take me. I don't know how the river bends or where the rapids may be. Radiotherapy completed my treatment, but my journey isn't finished. My cancer seems to be gone, but who can be sure? There are no curtainities, and from time to time a new pain has panicked myself and my loved ones. My body may be healed now but adjusting to the changes in my life and the recovery of my emotions, my soul, and my spirit takes longer.'

Image and poem reproduced with permission of Michele Petrone

A little bit of history: some key players

KEY POINTS

◆ Good care of the dying has always been regarded by the medical establishment as a key part of a doctor's duties.

◆ The standard of teaching provided on the subject has been of concern for a long time!

Perhaps it is that each era of history or each generation of doctors has its champions of the care of the dying. Hippocrates was, of course, a great orator on the subject, and in the Victorian era, when the medical profession in the UK was really beginning to shape itself, Sir Henry Halford (president of the Royal College of Physicians from 1820 until his death 24 years later) and William Munk were leading proponents. In his book published in 1887 entitled *Euthanasia: or medical treatment in aid of an easy death*, Munk writes:

> There is little to be found in medical writing on the management of the dying, or on the treatment best adapted to the relief of the sufferings incident to that condition. The subject is not specifically taught in any of our medical schools; and the young physician entering on the active duties of his office has to learn for himself, as best he may, what to do, and what not to do, in the most solemn and delicate position in which he can be placed – in the attendance of the dying, and administering the resources of the medical art, in aid of an easy, gentle, and placid death.

In spite of the advent of the new therapeutics in the twentieth century, the importance of the role of the doctor in the care of the dying changed little since Henry Halford's day, and had maybe become an even lower priority until very recently. What is more, doctors in the mid twentieth century became fearful of using opioids for pain relief because of the perceived risk of addiction.

This generation's pioneers

KEY POINT

In 1988 palliative medicine became a speciality recognized by the Royal College of Physicians, just like other specialities such as cardiology or neurology.

In the 1960s two new champions of the care of dying emerged. Cicely Saunders founded St Christopher's Hospice in London in 1967 and established that regular giving of morphine to patients with cancer pain achieved excellent control of pain for the vast majority of people with no risk of addiction whatsoever. Dame Cicely also re-established a philosophy of medicine that had been in danger of disappearing, that patients in all their aspects and dimensions, are the concern of the doctor, not the disease alone[2] (see Chapter 3).

Elizabeth Kubler-Ross, an American psychiatrist, has opened our minds to understanding the experiences of people who live with the knowledge that they will be dying in the near future. Her models of loss are fundamental to the way we have learnt to provide support to patients and families[3] (see Chapter 3). Psychiatrists in the UK, Colin Murray Parkes and John Hinton, have made an enormous contribution to the success of our work with patients and with bereaved families, and established how important care of the bereaved is in promoting physical and mental health.[4,5]

Epidemiology for the houseman

- Most people wish to die at home, but
- over 60% of people in the UK die in hospital;
- 10–15% of hospital beds are at any one point in time used for the care of patients with advanced disease;
- one-third of patients with advanced illness will die within a week of their final admission, but 40% will be in hospital for longer than 1 month;
- most hospital resources are used for people who are in the last year of their lives.

As a houseman then you will see a lot of people in hospital who have advanced disease, some of whom you will be caring for when they die. Figure 1.1 indicates the proportion of people dying from the common causes of death. In your first year as a doctor you will care for perhaps 40 people who will die in hospital. So you are likely to care for about 10 people who die from cancer; 18 people who die from heart attacks, chronic heart disease, or stroke; and 4 people

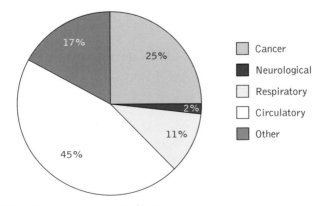

Fig. 1.1 What diseases do people die from?

who die from respiratory causes. This will, of course, be influenced by the speciality of the wards you work on.

Remember, however, that you'll be looking after at least three times this number of people who have advanced disease, are perhaps in the last 6 months of their life, but aren't dying during this admission.

How to care well for the dying
What do patients and their carers need?

CASE HISTORY EXERCISE

Mrs Ada Jones is a 62-year-old lady. She lives with John to whom she has been married for 5 years. She was divorced from Fred 10 years ago. They had four children together. John has two children from his previous marriage. Ada and John have 14 grandchildren and two great-grandchildren. She works as a dinner lady at the local primary school. She was diagnosed with motor neurone disease 6 months ago and is now unable to walk. She has asked her GP to visit today because she has found that she is coughing when swallowing drinks.

◆ What do you think might be on Mrs Jones's mind?

◆ What do you think Mrs Jones might want from her GP?

◆ What do you think the GP will be wanting to think about with her?

(see our thoughts p. 11)

LEARNING EXERCISE

If you would like to know more about living and dying with MND,

◆ read *Motor neurone disease*[6]

◆ search the web; good places to start are: www.mndassociation.org and www.home.vicnet.net.au/~mndaust

Perhaps another patient may be thinking

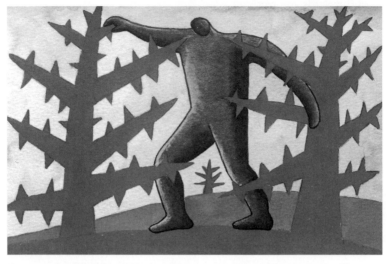

1.4 The pain of it all. 'So now I have a diagnosis. Hodgkin's disease.. Let's call it cancer.
I've heard of that. I know what it is – Fiona, a woman I live with is having chemotherapy
for breast cancer. This is different, I'm told. They don't tell you that an 80% chance of
cure means a 20% chance of death. You're left to work that one out for yourself. Death.
Life is bad enough, that's what I thought. But who do I tell? Mum, I want to die. Hey,
lover of mine, I think forever might be closer than I thought. Hi good friend, want to
talk about euthanasia and writing a will?

'We're all in pain, why can't we share our pain?'

Death and illness are almost taboo subjects even though we will all die eventually. Who isn't
frightened and doesn't find it difficult to talk to someone they know might be dying? I was-
n't prepared, neither were my family and friends. Who's going to help me, listen to me,
understand me, be there for me – just for me. Not be frightened by my thoughts and feelings of having my life threatened, changed, and maybe dying at the end of it all anyway.

Image and poems reproduced with permission of Michele Petrone

The good doctor's essential toolkit

Good medical practice, in whatever speciality field, integrates knowledge,
skills, and attitudes. Unfortunately, we have seen many sad examples that have
been taken before the General Medical Council (GMC) where only one aspect
of this triad has been practised by doctors, to the cost of the patient. All three
components are important for you to develop to provide good palliative care for
your patients. For example:

1. You will need to KNOW
   - about diseases and their natural history,
   - about drugs and their safe use,
   - about palliative care services and how to access them.

2. You will need to be SKILLED in

- communication,
- various technical procedures, such as aspiration of ascites.

3. In your ATTITUDE to patients you should be

- empathetic,
- holistic.

In Appendix 1 we have formatted the curriculum for medical students developed by the Association for Palliative Medicine of Great Britain and Ireland as a tool for you to use to reflect on what currently you know and feel confident in about your abilities, and to have a clear understanding of what you need to develop. Perhaps you could fill in this questionnaire before reading this book and then repeat it afterwards to see how much you've learnt.

> **KEY POINT**
>
> In essence, patients and their carers may need:
>
> - listening to their concerns
> - information and discussion
> - support and counselling
> - symptom control
> - continuity of care and good team work
> - access to expert services
> - practical help.

> **SUMMARY BOX**
>
> Whichever branch of medicine you choose to specialize in, you will be caring for people affected by advanced and terminal diseases. Patients with incurable illness can be professionally and personally challenging. Your professional competence in palliative care is not optional. The curriculum defined by the Association for Palliative Medicine will guide you in obtaining the appropriate knowledge skills and attitudes that will enable you to provide good care and gain a great deal of professional satisfaction.

Case history exercise: some thoughts on Mrs Jones

Of course we can only guess what is on Mrs Jones's mind and what she might want from us as her doctor. Only when we ask her will we really find out. Having some thoughts, however, will help you prepare for such a consultation, both in thinking about the answers but also in asking open questions that will help her tell you what she is thinking and feeling. We usually use empathy (putting ourselves in her situation) to guess what might be on her mind, but we can also use the evidence base to guide us (i.e. what patients have told us in the past or told researchers) without, of course, making foolhardy assumptions for the individual patient.

Mrs Jones will probably want to know

- what is happening to cause the swallowing problems;
- what it means about the progress of the MND;
- what can be done to improve things.

She will probably want her doctor to discuss with her

- the treatment options;
- the detail of what they entail;
- the choices she can make.

She might want

- to know how long her prognosis is;
- to know what she can expect to happen from now;
- to talk about telling her family and the impact of her diagnosis and deterioration on them.

Her doctor might want

- to learn more about her thoughts about decisions around the end of life, such as the use of antibiotics for pneumonia;
- to review the practical help that is needed and the arrangements for anticipating problems and preventing crises.

It is unlikely that the GP has much experience of MND and may wish to gain expert advice and support from the MND Association and the local palliative care service and specialist MND nurses.

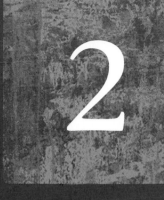

CHAPTER 2

Taking a palliative care history and handling difficult situations

- ◆ Introduction *15*
- ◆ Taking a palliative care history: the patient's story *15*
- ◆ A focused examination and investigation *20*
- ◆ Barriers and blocking *21*
- ◆ Handling difficult situations *22*
- ◆ Limited communication: another challenge *23*
- ◆ Real-world history taking *25*

CHAPTER 2

Taking a palliative care history and handling difficult situations

Introduction

At the risk of stating the blindingly obvious, making an accurate assessment of our patients' needs, knowing the best management options, and involving patients and carers in decision making are the key tasks of being a good doctor. The bedrock for our success in this process is our ability to communicate. Dealing with patients with life-threatening illnesses also raises the possibility of you having to handle difficult questions and situations (see box). Patients come to us seeking help; they have questions that need answering. We have to answer them well.

> **Some tricky situations**
>
> 'Is it serious?'
> 'How long have I got?'
> 'Don't tell him he's dying, it'll kill him'
> 'Why can't he be cured?'
> 'Can you end it for me?'

If you ask patients about how well doctors communicate, you will get a mixed response. Many doctors will get rave reviews, where as others have obviously damaged patients emotionally. No one sets out to be a bad communicator, and we all run the risk of underperforming from time to time. All we can do is continually work at getting it right as often as possible—this is no small task.

Taking a palliative care history: the patient's story

To the novice student medicine is magical. The skilled professional asks questions, lays on hands and applies some mysterious technology, and 'hey presto' a diagnosis. Indeed, diagnostic revelations are highly prized by the profession; the more obscure the better. However, medicine in general, and palliative care specifically, does not stop there. Not only is there treatment to consider, but future complications should be anticipated and you will need the same precise skills to diagnose them accurately. Also, palliative care actively goes beyond the physical and seeks to ease the psychological, social, and spiritual needs of patients (see Chapter 3).

To become skilled in history taking takes practice. The received wisdom in medical training is for you to see as many patients as possible—practice makes perfect. This is true, but what it fails to recognize is that, without thinking about what we are doing, we are likely to fall into bad habits or not develop good ones. And it is unusual for us to have many opportunities to reflect and learn about consulting. Taking a history has many facets and subtleties that need to be learnt. Understandably, many communication skills teaching sessions, focus rather more on dramatic scenarios (e.g. breaking bad news, the angry patient, etc.), yet there is more to learn than this. This section aims to give you some tips on taking a good history from the patients that we, as students and doctors, see each and every day. There is a lot written on this, but what we give you here is a flavour of some of the important considerations.

Listening and talking

As medical students we are generally taught to take a history by asking a series of specific questions in a structured format. Using conventions like this can be really helpful—we all know what is expected of us and where to find things in the notes. I certainly remember nervously referring to my checklist of questions, fearful that if I didn't ask all the questions then my ignorance would be revealed on the next teaching ward round. Truly terrifying! I was concerned with how I would appear rather than whether I had made the fullest assessment of the patient.

However, as you've noticed, patients don't give their history according to our conventions and checklists, but give you information in a way that makes sense to them. They are not trying to be awkward, even if it feels like that to you. One way of getting round this problem is for you to take charge by interrupting them and asking your questions anyway. Sure, you would have series of things to write in the notes, but what would you have found out? Probably the bare minimum.

Alternatively you could ask a good opening question and let the patient tell their story. As the consultation proceeds you can then seek clarification and attempt to explain things in a way that makes sense to the patient (see

> **THINK POINT**
>
> Did you know that on average the doctor interrupts the patient within 18 seconds of the consultation starting?

> **THINK POINT**
>
> Did you know that on average 54% of patients' problems are not elicited during the consultation?

Learning exercise). This will mean that the patient does more of the talking initially, then you start to say more as the consultation goes on (see Fig. 2.1).

> **LEARNING EXERCISE** Trying it out!
>
> For the next patient you have to clerk, let the consultation flow and keep your writing to a minimum. Then write your history up in full afterwards. See what sort of information you get.

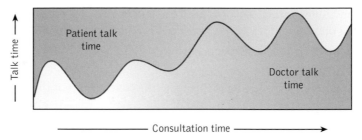

Fig. 2.1 Rough representation of the time spent talking by the patient and the doctor during a consultation

There is evidence that this approach works, you tend to get better-quality information, you understand patients more holistically, and it actually takes no longer than if you were going through your checklist anyway.

Doing this can feel a bit scary at first. 'But what if I dry up or forget to ask the really important question?' In fact, it is far easier than you would think. It feels more natural and you will find yourself asking all the important questions anyway, especially the questions most relevant to the patient. It should feel more like a 'purposeful discussion' and less like an interrogation. Below are a few tips on how to do this:

- Use open questions to get patients talking and closed ones if you need to clarify something (see Table 2.1).

- Give the impression that you can give them time or actually create time to talk.

- Use non-verbal communication techniques to enhance disclosure and rapport (e.g. sitting not standing, good eye contact, nodding the head, etc.).

- Make sure no one can overhear you. It is important to respect privacy and ensure that confidentiality is maintained as much as possible.

- Be happy for information to come in any order the patient gives it.

- Have a clear framework for a history in your head so that you can assimilate information as it is given without interrupting and stopping the patient's flow (see Think point). You should write it in the standard convention afterwards.

- Get the patient to expand on a subject by making encouraging noises (e.g. 'I see,'

LEARNING EXERCISE

When you next sit in on a consultation, note whether the doctor is asking open or closed questions, and see what sort of information they generate.

THINK POINT
Getting the whole picture

Think of history taking as rather like a jigsaw. The pieces come to you at random, and the overall picture seems a muddled at first, but as you go on, putting bits together, the true picture emerges.

'Mmm'), summarizing what has just been said to you, or reflecting back (e.g. so your doctor said …). In the jargon this is called active listening.

- Listen carefully to what patients say, the key to their problems are in the words they use.
- Be comfortable with letting the patient take control, even if this means them getting upset.

Table 2.1 Examples of open and closed questions

Examples of open questions	Examples of closed questions
'How are you today?'	'When did you have your endoscopy?'
'How can I help you?'	'Where exactly is your pain?'
'Tell me about your illness.'	'Would you say that you feel sick at meal times?'
'Tell me about your pain.'	'Are you worried about your wife?'
'You seem worried to me.'	'Do you take your tablet regularly?'
'Is there anything you want to ask me?'	'Can I talk about that at the next appointment?'

Attention to detail

Patients facing a terminal illness can have a wide range of complex problems. In order to manage them effectively you need to be precise. For instance, a patient's pain needs to be clearly defined. The same attention to detail should also be given to other symptoms, and equal precision is needed for the more psychosocial problems. Misunderstandings or assumptions made when taking an initial history will lead to you making mistakes.

Often a family tree can really help in giving you a clear idea of all the key players, or lack of them, in a patients life (see box).

One useful way of recording information is to write actual quotes in the notes. For instance, compare 'Paracetamol stopped' to 'Those paracetamol were no bloody good—I stopped them!' Both statements could be a record of the same event, but consider how much more information the second one gives you.

Normally the psychosocial component of a medical history tends to be relegated to perhaps a few comments about occupation and carers at home. As this book demonstrates, in palliative care this is rarely enough. You need to make it your business to explore all those issues that are important to the patient. This does not mean being nosy, but giving patients the chance to express themselves and for you to take this seriously (see Chapter 3).

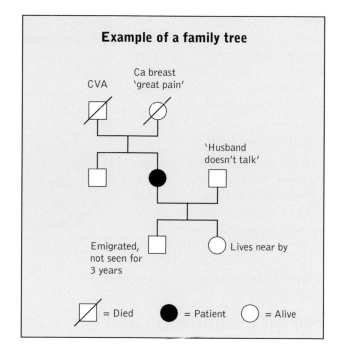

Example of a family tree

Without such attention to detail, you will have your work cut out to be as effective a doctor.

The problem list

The 'standard' medical history ends with the most likely diagnosis and its differential. As we have already emphasized, in palliative medicine we are interested in far more than this. Any problem, however trivial it might seem to you, deserves your attention. We might not be able to 'cure' it as such, but there is always something you can do to ease it, even if it is listening and understanding.

The problem list is a useful way of recording all the patient's problems (see box). It allows you to consider systematically your approach to each of them independently and to review them at a future date. Also, if you get into the habit of writing all the problems down, you are less likely to overlook difficul-

THINK POINT Patient lists—friend or foe?

Most doctors will tell you of their irritation of being presented with a list of problems by a patient. 'They take so long'. But think about it; we spend all this time trying to understand what patients really want, so really a patient list is something to be celebrated! A patient list is their agenda—a history is ours.

ties you could do something about. Under each problem you can outline your proposed plan of action, be it drugs, referral to another member of the team, a subject for discussion next time, or something you need to get advice from someone else about.

Summarizing

During, and especially at the end of, the consultation it is useful to summarize to the patient what was said and what you have agreed is going to happen next. This tells the patient that you have been listening, shows that you want to get it right, allows the patient to correct any misunderstanding, gives an opportunity for shared planning, and helps recall.

> **PROBLEM LIST**
>
> An example of a problem list:
>
> 1. Shortness of breath
> 2. Pain
> 3. Anxiety for the future
> 4. Husband's inability to talk about cancer
> 5. Son living in Australia
> 6. Loss of role (work)
> 7. Tablet sceptic

A focused examination and investigation

As medical students we are taught to do 'a full examination.' In part this is designed to get us to practise our new-found examination skills—which is really useful. However, if we do it without thinking, we often fail to make links with the history and therefore come to wrong conclusions. It is also important to respect patient autonomy and dignity by not examining for the sake of it, especially when the patient is frail and vulnerable, which is often the case in palliative care. It is best to think before you examine, 'How will my findings influence my management.' If in doubt, examine, but if the honest answer is 'Not at all,' then it is best to omit this aspect of the examination.

The same principle of thinking and justifying to yourself also applies when ordering investigations. The temptation to perform 'routine bloods' on all patients admitted should be resisted. Ask yourself, 'How is this test going to help me help my patient?' Investigate patients if it is in their best interest, but

> **THINK POINT** What examination to do and test to order?
>
> Think:
>
> ◆ What hypotheses have I formed during the history?
> ◆ What examination or investigation would confirm or disconfirm my hypotheses?
> ◆ What are the important associated things I need to check?

not if it is in your best interest (i.e. so you look good on the next ward round!). This can be difficult in some hospital teams, but if you can explain your principles, most clinicians should respect this.

Barriers and blocking

Taking a good history and handling difficult situations are challenges to us all. The minute you think you are good at it is the time when you are probably underperforming. A challenging situation can make us want to use our power in the consultation to 'close patients down' so we keep control of the consultation (see box).

Much research has been done in this area, but perhaps the work by Maguire and Faulkner is the most celebrated.[1] They categorized various blocking techniques used by doctors and nurses:

- Behaving all 'doctor like' and aloof, e.g. standing up in your white coat, avoiding eye contact, and talking to the nurse.
- Getting into small talk.
- Ignoring patients' questions.
- Dealing only with the positive, 'Don't worry about that, at least you're going home today'.
- False or premature reassurance, saying it will be 'alright' when it is obvious to all that it won't.

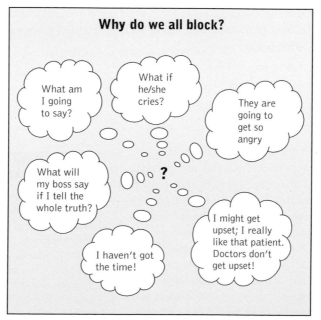

Why do we all block?

What am I going to say?

What if he/she cries?

They are going to get so angry

What will my boss say if I tell the whole truth?

I haven't got the time!

I might get upset; I really like that patient. Doctors don't get upset!

- Switching the topic: patient: 'Am I dying?', doctor: 'How is your breathing today?'.
- Passing the buck: 'I don't know, you better ask the consultant,' when the consultant is not going to see the patient until outpatients in 2 weeks' time and you know the answer anyway.
- Use of jargon—patient: 'Is it cancer?'; doctor: 'You've got an adenocarcinoma of the right main bronchus'.

The shocking truth is that all of us will use these techniques regularly, most of the time without knowing it. The best we can do is to be aware of them and be mindful of the sort of situations when we might use them. In this way you can limit the damage caused by blocking.

LEARNING EXERCISE

Write these blocking techniques down and watch a doctor consult. See if he or she uses any of them. Perhaps you could discuss this with the doctor you observe.

Handling difficult situations

General principles

Much of what we've talked about so far applies equally in more difficult situations, only the emotion, and therefore the stakes, tend to be higher in the circumstances listed below:

- breaking bad news
- giving a poor prognosis
- being asked to lie to patients
- the angry patient/family
- the request for euthanasia.

There are other situations that are also challenging, but these are the ones that tend to give students and doctors alike most anxiety. Much of our success in these sorts of consultations depends on our sensitivity and confidence. A textbook like this cannot teach these skills, all we can do is to give you some guidance. That is not to say that these skills cannot be learnt—they can. All readers will have an opportunity to have communication

---

THINK POINT

Did you know that 60% of doctors felt that in retrospect their undergraduate communication skills training was 'really helpful', yet at the time only 30% did? Why?

> ### Real quotes from doctors about breaking bad news
>
> 'It's probably the most important clinical thing I do. Its got to set the framework for the treatment.'
>
> 'If the patient has been alive for 50 years, they don't need to be told they're dying in a minute.'

skills training, either by role play or video work. We urge you to take these opportunities, even if you really feel uncomfortable about it.

Your approach to these problems will be unique to you and the particular situation. In general, however, such consultations work best when they follow the pattern outlined in the Fig. 2.2. Not that communication is ever this structured—thank goodness! However, the direction tends to follow these moves.

We can't, of course, be there to tell you what words to use, or consider the infinite number of possible variations on these themes. All we can say is that you will be in these positions, that how you do it makes a difference, and that it is never easy.

Limited communication: another challenge

All the above assumes that the patient can enter into open discussion. In some circumstances this is not the case, either because the patient:

- is too ill;
- is unconscious or dying;
- doesn't share a common language/culture with the doctor;
- does not wish to discuss the issues you want to cover.

In all such situations communication will, of course, be compromised. But it is still beholden on you to make every effort to overcome these problems, accepting, of course, that you should respect a patient's wish to avoid talking about certain topics. In many cases, a barrier to open communication means using others to fill in the gaps (e.g. carers, interpreters, other professionals). In so doing you have to make judgements as to the strength and validity of advocacy of each of these sources. This often means asking more than one person for

> ### LEARNING POINT
>
> When you are next talking to a patient who has been given bad news, ask how it was done and what felt like to him.

Getting ready	Whatever the scenario, think about the following:
	• is the setting conducive to open discussion?
	• have you got your facts right?
	• might the patient/family want someone with them?
	Be prepared to take time, be ready to observe and experience strong emotion and, above all, be as honest and as open as possible.

	Breaking bad news	Giving a poor prognosis	Being asked to lie to patients	The angry patient/family	Request for euthanasia
Getting them talking—ask open questions, use your silence	Get them to tell you their understanding of things. Summarize and clarify events so far	Check if anyone has told them before, why are they asking this now? Is it that they want to know what death is like?	Relatives can ask you to conceal information. Get them to tell you why they want you to do this	Let them talk, don't react, reflect their emotion back to them: 'This obviously has made you very angry'	Ask them what has made them come to ask you for euthanasia
Sense what they might be feeling/ thinking and respond accordingly–listen, pick up on cues, respond with open questions	Get a feel for their readiness to know, give them clues that it's bad news, let them deny if they want to	What are their hopes and are they realistic? Is there a particular date coming up (e.g. family wedding)	Get a clear understanding of their fears behind this request. Foster their trust	Try and understand their anger and validate it if you can. Make sure they feel heard	Try to understand the reason for this request. Is it a mark of distress or a calculated choice?
Share information —use appropriate language, check understanding, don't dominate	If ready to know, then tell them sensitively and at their pace. Give them plenty of space to think and ask questions, maintain hope	Be honest that you can't say for sure. Use their recent health as a means of justifying your opinion. Use loose terms (e.g. 'days or weeks')	Let them know that you understand their reasons but equally you can't lie to patients. Try and reassure that most patients know	If there has been a misunderstanding, apologize and try to explain this calmly. If they are just frightened—appreciate this	Explain that you cannot perform euthanasia. Try and answer the distress behind the request
What have they to expect next?	Don't overload them, tell them about support and when you can see them next, summarize	Summarize what you have discussed and let them know when they can speak to you again	Let the relatives know that, although you won't force information on the patient, you will have to tell if asked.	Summarize and make sure they feel understood. Offer a follow up meeting or an opportunity to speak to whoever they want	Summarize and let them know when you will see them again

Fig. 2.2 Handling tricky consultations

their input. This will confirm the impression you come to, so that you and your team can continue to act in the patient's best interest (see Chapter 4).

For those patients who do not share a common language with their doctor, the problem of communication is often complicated by cultural misunderstandings. Although familiarity with different cultural health beliefs might give us an advantage in understanding patients of a different ethnic group, we must be careful not to make assumptions about a patient's beliefs because of his or her cultural appearance. It might take time and effort, but we must understand and act in the best interests of all our patients. Below are some core skills in this area:

- Check on the pronunciation of your patient's name and how he or she wishes to be addressed.
- Discover patients' ideas, concerns, and expectations. That means listening to what they say.
- Be non-judgemental about ideas and beliefs.
- Demonstrate interest, concern, and respect.
- Behave with sensitivity throughout the physical examination.
- Incorporate their health understanding in your explanations.
- Have a negotiating approach to management.

Real-world history taking

Some would say that it is wrong to expect doctors to consult in the way outlined in this chapter all the time; either because it seems unnecessary as the issues are straightforward or because workload makes it impossible. However, it is important to:

- have an array of consultation skills at your fingertips that you trust and can call upon as needed
- know when to use different skills in different situations
- be able to recognize when your approach is not working, and know how to change to a more effective style.

SUMMARY BOX

◆ Taking a good history is central to good medical practice—there are useful tools for doing this well.

◆ Physical examination and investigations should always be done with thought and not by rote.

◆ Don't underestimate our ability to block open communication.

◆ There are useful ways of handling difficult situations (e.g. breaking bad news).

◆ Good communication is not an optional extra. You can learn to communicate well.

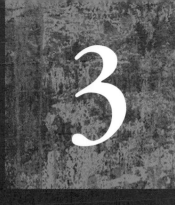

3

CHAPTER 3

Psychosocial aspects of palliative care, and why they matter

- Introduction *29*

- What actually are the psychosocial needs of dying patients and their families? *31*

- Scientific theory and how it helps *33*

- Learning to communicate effectively with patients and how it helps *37*

- Barriers to good psychosocial care, or what stops doctors being caring human beings *38*

CHAPTER 3

Psychosocial aspects of palliative care, and why they matter

A Physician is obligated to consider more than the diseased organ, more even than the whole man—he must view the man in his world

Harvey Cushing (1869–1939; of Cushing's disease fame)

Introduction

Medicine is about both understanding illness and understanding people. Each aspect is vitally important if we want to be good doctors. However, our training concentrates on the necessity of mastering the complexity of disease and the array of technical skills we can utilize; this is also what we tend to get taught and examined on. What is more, we soon find that this is what can amaze and amuse our friends (see Think point). However, this emphasis makes it harder to always see the value in considering the wider context of the disease experience for our patients.

> **THINK POINT**
>
> Recognizing a Graham Steele murmur on the patient in bed 12 and getting your patient to tell you what was really terrifying him or her are both highly skilled jobs you could do. But which sounds the more impressive, and why?

An impending death, like almost no other situation in medicine, reminds us of the importance of understanding people at the same time as we manage their disease (see Learning exercise).

Did you know that if you can appreciate the patient's perspective when he or she is ill, you are:

- more likely to be effective at making accurate assessments of patients;
- more likely to succeed in controlling patients' physical symptoms (see Chapter 5);
- more like to feel that the patient values your help; one of the most positive rewards in practising medicine;
- more likely to diagnose and treat depression;

LEARNING EXERCISE The challenge—it's about you

You can do this on your own or with a fellow student.

1. Write down all the things that are important in your life (e.g. family, friends, your hopes for the future, etc.).

2. Now imagine you were told that you had a diagnosis, the average prognosis of which was 12 months.

3. Cross off the list the things you will not be able to do and imagine (or tell your friend) what that feels like. How you would want health professionals to help you?

LEARNING EXERCISE What do patients want from you?

When you next see a patient and you have the time, try asking the following (it can be any patient):

♦ Which doctors have you found most helpful?

♦ Why were they good at their job?

♦ Which doctors have not been as helpful (no names!)?

♦ What was it that made them less helpful?

♦ What do they think a doctor should be like when looking after someone who is dying?

● less likely to make mistakes and have complaints made about you;

● less likely to feel burnt out; and increasingly be;

● more likely to pass exams! More and more exams are expecting students to demonstrate their appreciation of the psychosocial aspects of medicine.

For some, this chapter will be inherently interesting, we hope you enjoy it. To the more sceptical, we challenge you to read it, and answer yourself this question: 'What sort of doctor will your dying patients need?' (see Learning exercise 'What do patients want from you?').

So how can I improve?

Developing our attitude in this area is a life-long task for us all. We need to be able to constantly reflect and learn from our experience and strive to be better doctors as a consequence (easier said than done). How we each do this depends on many influences, and one chapter in one book can only hope to have a

THINK POINT

In a recent survey, 79% of house officers said they felt uncomfortable dealing with patient's psychosocial needs—will you?

very modest effect. However, we hope that we can give you an introduction to some of the methods and ways of thinking that could help you to be a more effective doctor in understanding patients.

What actually are the psychosocial needs of dying patients and their families?

This case history is but one patient's story and illustrates the extent of the psychosocial needs of patients who are dying. Of course, each patient you look after will have his or her own story and resulting needs. We must strive to understand how they and their families are feeling. On the face of it this seems complex. However, some emotions can be reasonably predicted and should be considered when interviewing patients; namely, fear, sadness, and anger (see Fig. 3.1).

Figure 3.1 also illustrates some of the aspects of life considered important by most of us; the very things that make us tick. It is how each patient views and copes with each of these components when facing the end of their life, that drives their emotions and subsequent behaviour. At the same time as the patient is tussling with such thoughts, his or her relatives and friends are likely to be concerned about similar issues.

Understanding what is important to patients and their families in the past, now, and in the future will give us a very clear idea of why they feel and behave as they do. Only then do we stand a chance of *really* helping them with their worries and concerns.

CASE HISTORY A true story

Colin was 54 when he died, 3 years after his diagnosis of renal cell carcinoma was made. He was a self-employed management consultant who had separated from Karen, because of several infidelities. She, however, was his main carer in his last months. He had three children; Judith, studying sports science; Claire, a nanny; and Joseph, who was doing his A levels. His mother lived alone and suffered from Alzheimer's disease.

Think about each of these characters and try to imagine the issues:

◆ Colin's views of his own, premature death; feeling about his relationship with Karen; and his thoughts about his mother.

◆ Karen's feelings about her relationship with Colin, her thoughts about her future role and responsibilities.

◆ The children's feelings about their father's death and his past infidelities.

It's little wonder many patients and their carers will be frightened and suffer as a consequence!

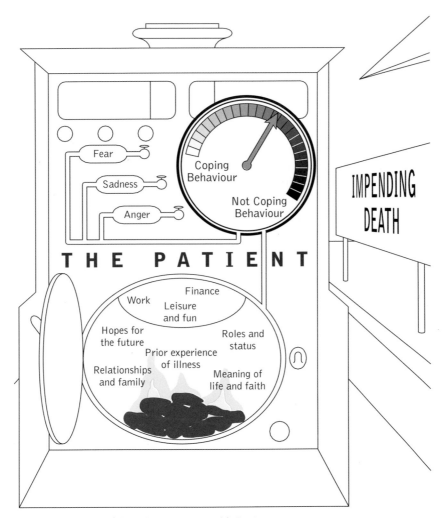

Fig. 3.1 The train of thought, emotion, and behaviour

We are all familiar with the emotions of sadness, fear, and anger, but few of us have felt these emotions in the same way as someone facing their own death. Patients differ in how they cope. Some take their impending death seemingly in their stride; others fluctuate in their ability to cope; and some struggle to retain any control. The forces that influence how patients cope are diverse to say the least. When speaking to patients we must give them an opportunity to express their feelings at a pace they are happy with. Learning to listen and making patients feel understood is a central skill of being an effective doctor. Not only will people feel so much better from being understood, you will probably find your work more rewarding (see Learning exercise). In Chapter 2 we out-

---

LEARNING EXERCISE What is it like to look after the dying?

Choose a senior colleague you respect and ask him or her the following sorts of questions:

◆ Can you remember the last dying patient you looked after, where things went well?

◆ What sort of person was the patient?

◆ When you were looking after the patient, how well did you understand what they wanted?

◆ What did it feel like to look after this patient?

After you've heard the answers, consider the depth at which the doctor knew the patient's psychosocial background.

---

lined some of the skills needed to explore these issues with patients in a way that is effective.

Scientific theory and how it helps

One way of helping us be effective in our understanding of the psychosocial needs of our patients, is to be familiar with some of the scientific theory that can explain what is going on (see Think point). If we are able to stand outside of the process and analyse it, then we can:

● make better sense of the emotions and behaviour we observe;

● feel that the consultation is not out of control and that the patient's emotions and behaviour do not overwhelm us;

● better predict what is going on and so be more effective in how we offer help.

THINK POINT Theories and holidays—an analogy to understanding

Imagine planning an exciting holiday to a place you're never visited. How would you find out about where you were going? You'd go to different sources to get the information; road map, globe, travel guide, the web, a well-travelled friend, etc. Each source would tell you something true about the place, albeit from slightly different perspectives. The same could be said for theories that explain patients' emotions and behaviour. Each theory gives us a clearer understanding of what is going on. No one theory gives us all the answers, and some are more useful than others in different circumstances. However, they can all help guide us as we try to make sense of our patients.

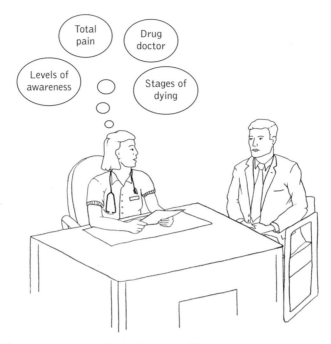

Fig. 3.2 Using theories and models in the real world

Different disciplines have contributed to our understanding of how patients' feelings and behaviour can be understood, (Fig. 3.2). There is a lot written on this subject and it is beyond the scope of this book to give you a very detailed account of all relevant theories. What we hope is that by showing you a sample of some of the most quoted work, you will be able to appreciate the effectiveness of this approach in everyday medical practice.

Stages of dying

In her often-quoted work, following her observations of dying patients, Kubler–Ross describes five stages of dying.[1] These stages may be experienced sequentially, with individuals moving from stage to stage. However, often patients tend to jump around the stages, back and forth. Some patients seem to reach 'acceptance' very quickly.

1. Denial: avoiding the harsh reality when given a terminal diagnosis.

2. Anger: the 'Why me?' response. The anger can be directed at family or friends, or at their doctor.

3. Bargaining: the patient attempts to ward off the inevitable by making a deal with the doctor, family, or God. 'Surely doctor, if I have this big operation I'm bound to be cured?'

4. Depression: the realization of the forthcoming loss of life results in feelings of depression, guilt, anxiety, and hopelessness.

5. Acceptance: the end of the struggle. The patient has generally transcended the previous four stages of emotional adaptation.

Total pain

Dame Cecily Saunders was the founder of the modern hospice movement in the UK, she also devised the concept of total pain.[2] Classically, pain is understood physiologically in terms of a noxious stimulus causing an unpleasant sensation; and this is true. However, it is also sometimes useful to view it more holistically (Fig. 3.3). A patient's pain will be worse if they also have to suffer powerful negative emotions, such as anxiety, anger, and depression. In fact, for those that struggle to express their distress, using the language of pain can be helpful. This concept of total pain can be useful when assessing patients whose pain presents atypically, or where the response to analgesics is inconsistent or incomplete. It is important not to dismiss this pain as unreal or 'in the mind', it isn't and must be taken seriously, requiring active management. Only, this management might not mean the escalation of analgesic drugs, but allowing the patient's distress to be recognized and understood, and, if appropriate, managed by non-pharmacological methods.

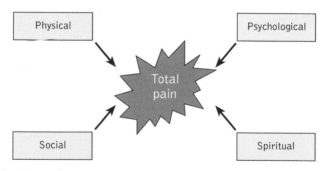

Fig. 3.3 The theory of total pain

Contexts of awareness

Glaser and Strauss[3] and later Timmermans,[4] have described patients' attitudes to the news of their impending death according to 'contexts of awareness'. It is believed that patients, and those important to them, can be categorized into one of the groups shown in Fig. 3.4.

Obviously the ideal position for the medical staff and most patients is active open awareness. Although all are emotionally exacting, this phase gives the greatest hope of the death the patient most wishes.

Contexts of awareness

Closed awareness	Suspended awareness	Mutual pretence	Open awareness
The patient does not recognize they are dying, but everyone else does.	The patient suspects what others know and attempts to verify this, but staff and family avoid the questioning.	All the players in the game (patient, family and staff) are aware of the impending death, but all continue as if they are not.	Everyone is aware of the impending death and this may be acknowledged in interactions.

Suspended open awareness	Uncertain awareness	Active open awareness
The truth is given but then blocked out by patients and their kin.	Patients and professionals selectively retain good information. Ignoring more pessimistic news. Medical uncertainty is used to draw a veil over the negatives.	The patient and family understand the prognosis and actively try to come to terms with it. The patient no longer hopes for recovery.

Fig. 3.4 Awareness of dying

Drug doctor

Putting aside the non-PC title of this book, Balint has been hugely influential.[5] His work in the late 1950s resulted in the concept of 'drug doctor'. He felt that one of the most frequently used and powerful agents within the consultation was the doctor. Patients can gain great benefit, or indeed great harm, from how the doctor interacts with them. This can be a useful concept to hold when speaking with patients, especially in those consultations when we do not seem to be doing anything but listen. You will be surprised how much being understood really helps.

LEARNING EXERCISE Theory and practice

Next time you're observing a doctor consult, especially in a challenging situation, see if any of the theories apply. When you are more skilled you may be able to think of some of these theories when listening to patients yourself. At the end ask yourself 'Does it help to think like this?'

Learning to communicate effectively with patients and how it helps

If we are to really understand what patients think and feel, we need to be skilled at getting them to share their psychosocial concerns with us. We have to be comfortable about taking a patient-centred history, talking about what worries them, and listening, and be able to observe emotional distress (see Chapter 2). Only then will we be able to make accurate assessments of patients' needs and perform the high-quality medicine to which we all aspire. What is more, inaccurate assessment not only cause patients to suffer; they waste time and resources and lead to complaints.

Some of the specific communications skills required in palliative care are covered in Chapter 2. However, communicating effectively with patients requires more than the knowledge of what you ought to say. It also requires you to have skills that need to be practised. Just to give you an idea of how important it is to get this right, have a look at what patients say (see box).

THINK POINT Two-minute warning

Did you know that if you spend the first 2 minutes of a consultation talking only about the patients' physical symptoms, they will assume you are interested in little else?

Quotes from real patients

'They were all very nice, very wonderful, but I realized afterwards that nobody told me anything.'

Female cancer patient

'He never told her the cancer was in her arm as well, but he told me and he said "I'll leave it with you to tell her."'

Husband of breast cancer patient

Whatever stage we are in our careers, we gain in experience as we see more and more patients. But this does not mean we necessarily get better at communicating. What we need to do is to be able to reflect on how we communicate in a way that promotes positive change. The easiest way of doing this is to take advantage of the increasing number of communication skills courses available. The most effective methods usually involve the rather scary business of being observed by your peers (either on video or in role play) and getting feedback from a skilled tutor. Most of us, especially as beginners in this sort of situation, find it intimidating. But it really will make a difference (see box).

Quotes about being taught communications skills

'My surgeon had been on one of those courses and he said he tried to encourage others to do so, but it seems that those who really need it don't *think* they need it.'

Female breast cancer patient

'I was not keen to do this at first, but found it really beneficial in the end.'

Medical student

'Role plays are always embarrassing, but always good.'

GP

Barriers to good psychosocial care, or what stops doctors being caring human beings

None of us wants to be unkind when dealing with patients, but all of us will be. Not all the time or at a level that causes significant distress, but it happens more than we might think. This is not because we want to be horrible, but because we are human. Only when we recognize this truth do we stand any chance of protecting our patients and ourselves from underperformance. By appreciating the pressures we are under and how we behave with patients, we can then develop ways of minimizing the damage.

External barriers

Our work environment has a significant impact on how we function as doctors. We have to deal with a range of pressures that can result in us not helping the dying as much as we would like or they would need. By recognizing these pressures we can go some way to anticipating when we might be underperforming:

- Workload and prioritization: it is little wonder that if we are required to work in a way that demands us to process patients at speed, then we run the risk of ignoring everything but the immediate and necessary. And rarely is the psychosocial considered immediate and necessary by professionals. Most of us, to a greater or lesser extent, fall foul of this most days. The danger is not recognizing it and developing a way of working that routinely excludes patients' psychosocial concerns.

- Colleagues: even if you have a well-developed appreciation of the importance of the psychosocial, but work with colleagues who don't share these views, then your efforts in this area can at best go unrewarded and at worst be openly criticized.

- Teamwork: good psychosocial care depends on team members collaborating in an atmosphere that promotes understanding of patients. If you work in a more isolated way, then opportunities to help patients will be missed.

- Place: for patients to tell us their worries, they need to feel confident and comfortable. Many of the places we are required to work are not conducive to such an atmosphere (e.g. a busy ward with little privacy).

Internal barriers

There are other barriers, closer to home, that might also stop us performing at our best. These include:

- Tiredness: if we are physically or emotionally exhausted then we may have little left to give to our patients. There is a paradox here; the more we give to our patients the higher the potential risk to our own emotional well being. What we obviously need to know is where the balance lies for us and when we are getting exhausted.

> **THINK POINT**
>
> To 'burn out' you've got to be alight in the first place, just as long as you don't make a complete ash of yourself!

- Work ethic: throughout our training we are rewarded for hard work. Taking a break or saying 'no' is considered by some as a sign of weakness and failure. All you have to ask yourself is; who are you failing if you get exhausted?

- Professional attitudes: some of our training leads us to believe that the psychosocial aspects of patient care are never our job. We're in this business to cure disease after all—aren't we? It is still possible to become a doctor and still truly believe this (we know *you* don't think like this!). Even when we are examined on attitude, it is possible to 'turn it on for the exam', but then, in practice, behave in way that reflects what we truly believe.

- Confidence: if you feel underconfident in how to help people with psychosocial problems, you may handle this by trying to ignore the issues. And given the power we have during the consultation, we are well able to avoid areas that make us uncomfortable. Hopefully, with experience and practice you should overcome this problem.

> **THINK POINTS**
>
> Does any of this sound like you:
> - Perfectionist
> - Overly conscientious
> - Like pleasing people
> - Need to control others
> - Great sense of responsibility
> - Chronic self-doubt
> - Uncomfortable with praise
>
> If so look out,
> BURNOUT ALERT

- Personal experience: doctors are people too! We will at some times in our lives

> **THINK POINT** Statistics on health risks for doctors
>
> As doctors we are said to be epidemiologically at an advantage for most diseases yet what does the following tell us about the work we do?
>
> | | Increased risk |
> | --- | --- |
> | Alcoholic cirrhosis | SMR 311 |
> | Depression | 28% of housemen are clinically depressed |
> | Suicide | SMR 172 male; |
> | | SMR 371 female |
>
> SMR = Standardized mortality ratio. 100 is the average rate and anything above 100 is an above-average rate.

undergo life events that stretch our coping strategies. This will affect our work to a greater or lesser degree. Sometimes, for instance after a loss and period of grief, we are in a better position to understand our patient's predicament. Conversely our emotional reserves can be stretched to the point where it is hard to accommodate the distress of others.

● Illness: our own physical or mental illness can also impact on how we behave as doctors. Do not underestimate this.

How to look after yourself—avoiding burnout

The statistics mentioned here (see box) should worry you. 'But it won't happen to me' we hear you say. You're probably right. But the truth is that we are all at risk. Failing to be aware of the rigours of our job and life makes us especially vulnerable to burnout. So how do we protect ourselves? The following will help:

● Recognizing when you are stressed and what makes you feel like this.

● Talk to colleagues. We all have a quick moan or share stories about difficult work situations. Doing this with someone who listens helps. You will be surprised how much of this goes on (see Learning exercise).

● Don't loose your sense of humour.

● Take breaks and learn how you best relax. Do something other than work.

● Learning to say no. Obviously we have a job of work to do and we aspire to do it to a high standard. And as professionals who are reasonably rewarded for what we do, we have at times to go the extra mile for our patients. However, this should not mean saying yes to extra tasks that are

LEARNING EXERCISE Doctors helping each other

Next time you're sitting in the doctors' mess, have a listen to what people are talking about.

♦ Are they listening to each other's worries?

♦ Are they being supportive?

not necessarily advantageous to our patients, or to us. You should not feel guilty about this.

● Plan whenever possible.

● Remember, how you work is in your own destiny. Medicine has the advantages of variety of work patterns; we have to be brave enough to choose the one we really want for ourselves.

SUMMARY BOX

♦ To do medicine, and especially palliative medicine, well, we need to be able to understand people as well as we understand their illness.

♦ Caring for people's psychosocial needs helps the dying patients far more than most doctors think.

♦ Patients' psychosocial needs are all those tings that make us all tick as people.

♦ Scientific theory helps us to understand people and their behaviour.

♦ Communicating effectively makes a difference and can be learnt.

♦ That are many things that stop well-meaning doctors performing at their best-look out for them.

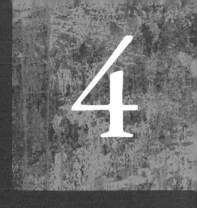

4

CHAPTER 4

Decisions around the end of life

◆ Death is a universal certainty *45*

◆ Advance statements about treatments *48*

◆ Doctor, I want to die: requests for euthanasia *50*

◆ Deciding when to stop life-sustaining treatments and when not to start them *51*

◆ Cardiopulmonary resuscitation *51*

◆ How can you help people die in the place of their choice? *55*

◆ Case history exercise: some thoughts on Mrs Collins *58*

◆ Case history exercise: some thoughts on Mrs Pierce *58*

Decisions around the end of life

The life story of every human being is a variation on the theme of loss through death—of every pet, every friend, every loved one, until sooner or later, the self, too, is taken. Yet this familiar companion on our journey remains a feared and hostile presence until the end; a Darth Vader, the dark assassin, who waits in the shadows until he cuts us down.

Kramer and Kramer (1993)[1]

Death is a universal certainty

There is nothing more certain than all our patients, all of us, will die one day, but unfortunately even for patients with advanced progressive illness the circumstances of death happen most often by default rather than by design. Doctors don't always recognize or acknowledge when a patient is nearing the end of his or her life. We may focus on the immediate problems caused by the illness and its threat to life. 'The treatment of a pulmonary embolus is …'. We may consider the need to relieve the distress caused by the physical symptoms, 'I'll give Mr Smith some diclofenac for the hip pain from his prostate cancer'. But how often do we take an overview of the whole situation; assess what has happened over the past weeks and months; find out what life has been like for the patient and their family; find out their views on how this illness episode should be managed? (See also Chapter 3.)

> *There may be doctors who in some sense are actually hiding death from themselves … Colluding in a an illusion with the sick people and their families, who really do believe that the next machine will keep their loved ones alive, against all hope. Doctors are obviously put in an extraordinarily difficult position in that it seems like a dereliction of their responsibilities if they don't make every effort to keep as many people alive as possible.*

Porter (1990)[2]

THINK POINTS

♦ The quality of care given to dying patients and communication with their relatives is one of the most common causes of complaint.

♦ Receiving a complaint is one of the most devastating experiences for doctors. We want to prevent both them and you having this experience.

♦ If you and your team don't consider that a patient may be dying, how will you provide them with the best care?

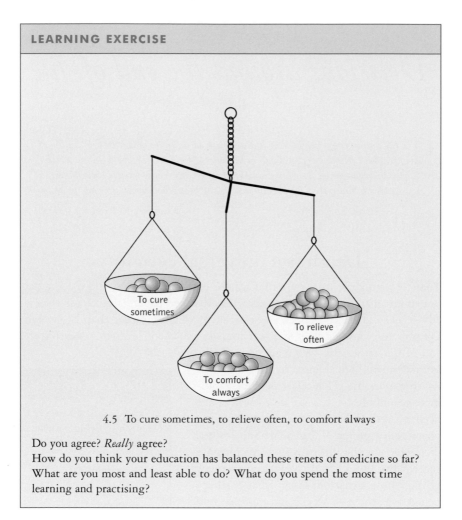

LEARNING EXERCISE

4.5 To cure sometimes, to relieve often, to comfort always

Do you agree? *Really* agree?
How do you think your education has balanced these tenets of medicine so far?
What are you most and least able to do? What do you spend the most time
learning and practising?

How can we hope to provide patients and their relatives with the best care
without recognizing and acknowledging that the patient is dying from his or
her illness?

A good death needs good decisions: what are the 'right' decisions for patients?

Decision making with patients with advanced progressive illnesses who may be
dying is complex. It is never black and white. We must decide what to do and
what not to do. We must resist the urge to undertake a medical intervention
without some evidence that it will be of help to the patient. We must weigh up

> **THINK POINT** Some tricky situations
>
> ◆ Is this treatment going to really help?
> ◆ It's so hard to know what the patient wants.
> ◆ Is it right to waste money on futile interventions?

the benefits and the adverse effects. In a situation which is often sad and, of course, unwanted, what seems most right for this patient? This is a grey art.

> **KEY POINTS** Further reading may be needed!
>
> Decision making is underpinned by the principles of medical ethics:
> ◆ beneficence,
> ◆ non-maleficence,
> ◆ justice,
> ◆ respect for autonomy.
>
> In reading this chapter you should call to mind these pillars of clinical judgment.
>
> If you haven't yet explored medical ethics, a good place to start is 'Medical ethics: four principles plus attention to scope'[3] and further reading is suggested at the end of the book.

However, there are some ethical principles, legal rulings, and evidence-based good practice that will help guide us to come to what is agreed as the best decision for that patient at that time.

> **CASE HISTORY EXERCISE**
>
> You have been called to see Mrs Collins who has severe Parkinson's disease. You've seen her three of four times this year. She has become progressively immobile and her husband tells you that she has been in bed for the past 2 weeks. They have called you because she has a painful and disturbing cough. You diagnose a severe lobar pneumonia. She is hypoxic, tachycardic, and hypotensive. You think she may die. You tell her she needs to be in hospital and her head 'goes down'. 'Do I have any choice doctor?' she asks.
>
> How will you take this further to make the best plan for Mrs Collins? What are the things you will need to discuss with her and her husband? Write short notes on the options in management of this lady. Think how the four ethical principles are at play here and how they will influence your decision.
>
> (see our thoughts on pp. 57–58.)

Patient autonomy: it is the patient's decisions, not ours

The patient's view on how their illness, life, and death should be managed is vital and their autonomy in this is generally of key ethical importance. In a patient who is able to talk to you and is competent then this relies on you communicating well with the patient, and providing them with high-quality information about the natural history of the condition and the likely benefits and potential problems of the treatments you are proposing. You need to inform patients accurately of their choices, in order for them to make decisions. Their choice is what counts, even if it differs from the choice of their family, our 'advice', or what may be considered 'normal'.

In a patient who is not competent, this decision making is more complex, but should be based as far as possible on the known wishes of the patient. Their autonomy is still of prime ethical importance when making decisions in their best interest.

KEY POINTS

A patient is judged competent to make a decision when they are:

◆ informed of the facts and probabilities;

◆ able to understand and believe the facts and probabilities;

◆ able to make a reasoned choice;

◆ able to communicate that choice.

The following may make the patient not competent to make a decision:

◆ reduced conscious state from injury, drugs, or infection;

◆ disorientation from mental illness;

◆ cerebral diseases, e.g. Alzheimer's;

◆ congenital mental disability;

◆ locked-in syndrome;

◆ coercion from others.

Advance statements about treatments

In recent years some patients have recorded their wishes, should they become incompetent, with respect to medical interventions in advance of those circumstances being reached. This advance statement is then available to guide clinicians when those circumstances arise. The BMA has drawn up guidance for good practice.[4] Advance statements can be:

● a statement of general beliefs and values;

- a requesting statement reflecting the individual's aspirations and preferences;
- a clear instruction refusing some or all medical procedures (advance directive);
- a statement that specifies a degree of irreversible impairment after which no life-sustaining treatment should be given;
- a statement that names a person who should be consulted about decisions.

Most of these statements are a guide to clinicians, but advance directives for refusal of treatment have legal force if made by a competent patient and they are applicable to the specific circumstances that have arisen. Advanced statements requesting clinical treatments which are at odds with clinical judgement about the patient's best interests do not have legal force.

People may choose to write advance statements in case something unexpected happens, for instance an accident that leads to the persistent vegetative state. More commonly, advance statements are written by people with progressive illnesses, to provide direction for circumstances that have a high likelihood of occurring. For this to be a competent decision patients need a lot of information and the opportunity for frank discussion. Some organization, such as the Motor Neurone Disease Association and the Terrence Higgins Trust, have developed particular information packs for people with MND and HIV, respectively.

In our experience, although some patients do write advance statements, many patients find that this is emotionally too difficult. It never seems quite the right time to address the likely and devastating future in black and white. Recording of more piecemeal discussions with patients concerning their general and specific views, is therefore important in helping the clinical team to make the best decisions when circumstances make the patient unable to guide us.

LEARNING EXERCISE

The next patient you see with a major stroke who can't communicate, think about:

- How do you know what decisions he or she would make about the treatments you think are and are not clinically appropriate?
- What are you basing these judgements on?
- How do you find out what the patient's wishes would be?

Then ask members of the team who are looking after the patient what their thoughts are and how they made decisions.

Doctor, I want to die: requests for euthanasia

Many patients will tell you that they want to die. A few will ask you to end it for them. How are you going to handle this? In the UK euthanasia is illegal, but a request to die demands more than simply a 'no-can-do' type response. It is clearly a very serious matter. It is often a sign of great distress, usually both physical and emotional, and it is also a sign that they feel they can trust you. Chapter 2 discusses the development of your communication skills in handling this situation. In our experience many, many patients feel this distressed but most do not request euthanasia. It is only when they trust you enough to listen, without disgust that they can share their distress of having to carry on living like this. For many patients the intensity of this feeling varies. Figure 4.1 indicates what may lie behind a request to die. Most of these issues can be resolved for most patients. Relieving a patient's distress is usually achievable, but often you will need help from a specialist palliative care team.

Euthanasia is a complex ethical, moral, and legal issue. To do it justice is beyond the scope of this text, and further reading is indicated at the end of the book.

> **THINK POINT**
>
> One study in a hospice service in The Netherlands has analysed the context of people's requests for euthanasia. Twenty to 30% of patients requested euthanasia at some point; 1.6% of patients actually left the hospice for euthanasia.

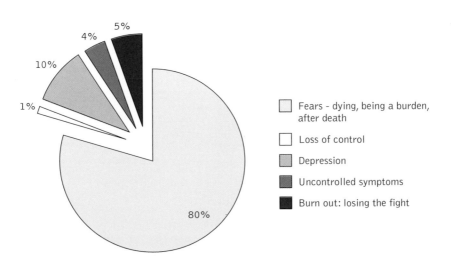

Fig. 4.1 Reasons why people may tell a doctor that they want to die

THINK POINT

We can not judge as external observers the circumstances that make suffering intolerable to any one individual. The young, bed-bound woman with every tube imaginable in place, with whom I sat and watched *East Enders* as Ethel asked Dot to help her die, told me she believed strongly in euthanasia, that we don't let dogs suffer like we do humans. 'Are you suffering?' I asked, expecting a very tricky conversation. 'Oh no. Life's OK' she said, to my amazement.

Deciding when to stop life-sustaining treatments and when not to start them

For people with advanced incurable progressive illness, the focus of their care is based on the quality of their lives. Doctors must weigh up carefully the appropriateness of use of active clinical measures that may prolong the length of life. The two key considerations are:

● Will they provide a good quality of life?

● Are they certain not to lengthen suffering?

All such decisions must be considered in a holistic context. For instance, will interventions possibly stop the patient going home?

A conscious patient may have clear views on what treatments they do and don't want, but can only make a competent decision if provided with information about the realistic benefits and adverse effects (see above). Only patients themselves can judge the quality of their lives.

For very sick patients who are not able to communicate their views on treatments and interventions, a framework for decision making is important (Figure 4.6).

In the dying patient hydration and nutrition are common issues of concerns to relatives and professionals that need to be thought through (see case history exercise on p. 53, and also refer to pp. 84–85). Table 4.1 indicates some of the considerations necessary in making the decision about the administration of parenteral fluids to a dying patient.

Cardiopulmonary resuscitation

Cardiopulmonary resuscitation (CPR) can be attempted on any individual in whom cardiac or respiratory function ceases. Of course, stopping breathing and the heart stopping happens as part of dying, and although CPR could theoretically be used on every individual prior to death this would seem inappropriate and deny the normality and certainty of death. The decision for each patient must be considered individually.

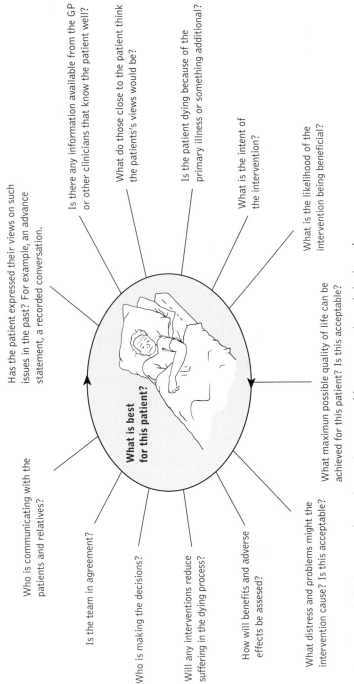

Has the patient expressed their views on such issues in the past? For example, an advance statement, a recorded conversation.

Is there any information available from the GP or other clinicians that know the patient well?

What do those close to the patient think the patients's views would be?

Is the patient dying because of the primary illness or something additional?

What is the intent of the intervention?

What is the likelihood of the intervention being beneficial?

What is best for this patient?

Who is communicating with the patients and relatives?

Is the team in agreement?

Who is making the decisions?

Will any interventions reduce suffering in the dying process?

How will benefits and adverse effects be assesed?

What distress and problems might the intervention cause? Is this acceptable?

What maximun possible quality of life can be achieved for this patient? Is this acceptable?

4.6 A framework for decision making when patients are unable to communicate their views about treatments

Table 4.1 Artificial hydration (IV fluids) during the dying phase: to use or not to use?

PROS	CONS
May reduce thirst in some patients (but good mouth care usually does as good a job)	May stop patients being at home
Seems less like we're just letting the patient die (but remember, he or she is dying from the disease not dehydration. Who are we treating really, us, the relatives, or the patient?)	May make death less 'natural', i.e. medicalized. Families may be less able to cuddle and get close with the pump/drip stand and infusion set getting in the way
May help circulation of drugs to relieve symptoms	May stop nurses giving mouth care
May reduce confusion	May cause pulmonary oedema
	May increase incontinence/restlessness from full bladder
	Venflons are painful and infusion sets constraining

CASE HISTORY EXERCISE

Mrs Pierce has had multiple sclerosis for 25 years. She has been admitted with a pneumonia. She is uable to communicate and she can not protect her airway when swallowing. You think that she may be dying. You need to consider whether you are going to:

◆ give her antibiotics;

◆ put up a drip;

◆ organize enteral feeding.

◆ attempt CPR.

Think how you might make these decisions. If you have a chance, discuss your thoughts with a doctor or senior nurse.

(see our thoughts on p. 58)

The key issues in considering whether resuscitation is appropriate for a patient with an advanced progressive disease are:

● does this patient want it?

● does cessation of cardiac and respiratory function represent the terminal event of that illness?

● is CPR likely to be effective or futile?

THINK POINT

In one study, nearly 50% of hospice inpatients with advanced cancer said they would definitely wish to be resuscitated if their heart stopped suddenly.

• what quality of life would CPR regain and what are the patient's views on this?

In hospital it is now good practice that the resuscitation status of all patients should be clear to all clinical staff. The responsibility for this lies with the patient's consultant. Each hospital you work in will have its own specific policy and you should be made aware of this during your induction.

In the community the issue is less medical-ized and good practice less clear.

The essence of making a good decision is in discussion: with the patient, with people close to them, and with the clinical team. This is obviously a sensitive area and your communication skills will need to be developed in this area.

THINK POINT

Further reading may be needed!
The success of resuscitation is vastly overestimated by patients. What is the success rate? See Ref. 5.

KEY POINTS

BMA guidelines: it is appropriate to consider a Do-Not-Resuscitate (DNR) decision in the following circumstances:

◆ where the patient's condition indicates that effective CPR is unlikely to be successful;

◆ where CPR is not in accord with the recorded, sustained wishes of the patient who is mentally competent;

◆ where CPR is not in accord with a valid and applicable advance directive;

◆ where successful CPR is likely to be followed by a length and quality of life which would not be in the best interests of the patient to sustain.

KEY POINTS

The entry in the medical records should:

◆ detail the decision;

◆ detail the reasons for the decision;

◆ detail the discussion leading to the decision;

◆ be signed with date and time;

◆ be communicated to the clinical team.

KEY POINTS

It is recommended best practice to always discuss the decision with the patient, but what if you have evidence to believe that it would be *detrimental* to the patient? If this is so perhaps you do not need to discuss the DNR decision when:

◆ a patient is judged incompetent;

◆ the DNR decision is being made on the grounds of futility;

◆ although CPR has a chance of success, the subsequent quality of life would not be in the patient's best interests;

◆ a patient indicates that they do not wish to discuss it.

This is controversial however and research indicates that, even though it is painful and worrying, more patients would like to be involved in these discussions than we currently approach. You will need to record your reasons for not discussing the decision with the patient in the notes.

You should always try and speak with relatives about the decision.

LEARNING EXERCISE

◆ Observe the process of making the decision with the next patient with an advanced, life-threatening illness admitted to your ward.

◆ Go with your medical team when they discuss CPR status with a patient and relatives.

◆ How are the nurses involved in the decision?

◆ Make sure that you are clear what, how, and where to write the decision in the patient's notes.

◆ Speak to the doctors and nurses about how they discuss these issues with the patient and the family.

◆ Remember that many teams do not always follow best practice. So if you see a decision made that does not follow the guidance given, that does not mean they have done it correctly.

How can you help people die in the place of their choice?

Most people say they would ideally wish to die at home. Theoretically, this should be achievable for those who die from progressive diseases, but it only happens for about one person in four. There has been much research into the reasons for this and the efficacy of interventions facilitating death at home.

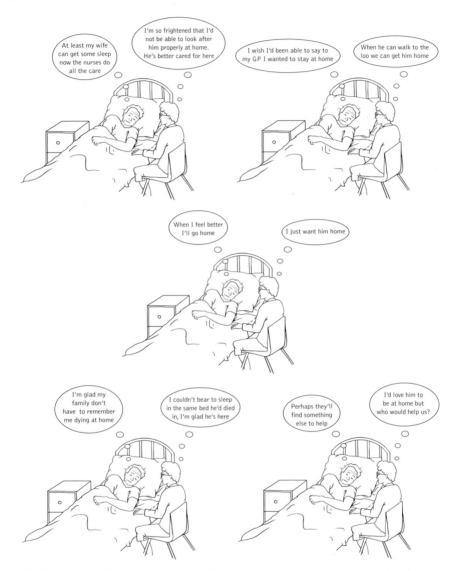

4.7 Helping people to die in the place of their choice requires that you try and understand their thoughts and fears

When it comes to it, not everyone will choose to die at home, but some of the research has implications for the way you can best work with patients and their families to help them achieve the best possible in their particular circumstances.

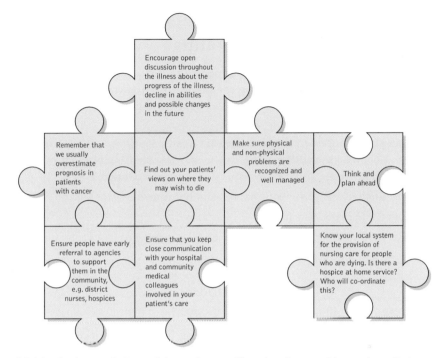

4.8 The fundamental pieces of the work you will need to do to enable people to die in the place of their choice

---

SUMMARY BOX

Decision making with and about people who are dying is complex. We have immense power as doctors which we have to use wisely to facilitate the best possible choices, decisions, and outcomes for patients. The ethical principals of autonomy, non-maleficence, beneficence, and justice underpin such decision making alongside the need for compassion, good communication, team working, and a sound knowledge of medico-legal and local clinical governance policies.

Everybody dies. The aim is to make it as good as possible for every individual. Finding out what this might mean for each person, and acting accordingly, is vital.

Case history exercise: some thoughts on Mrs Collins

Mrs Collins has given you a cue to explore this situation further with her. Before discussing the choices, open the discussion. You can't make the best plan until you understand all the components that should be considered. You will need to try and find out:

- What she is concerned about. Is she concerned about hospital, wanting to stay at home, not wanting active treatment, or something else? (It may well be something you can't guess at and you need to ask.)
- What are her thoughts about her life and her illness in general?
- What are her thoughts about her future care?
- Have you explained to her fully enough what you think is happening?
- Are there questions she wants to ask you?

The choices

There are four possible plans:

- To admit to hospital for intensive treatment. Would she/you consider ventilation as appropriate if it is clinically indicated?
- To admit to a GP unit/cottage hospital (if available). Is this to provide the nursing care she needs or the medical treatments? Does she need an X-ray, blood gases, or other hospital type support?
- To stay at home with extra nursing care, analgesia, oxygen, and antibiotics, started by you IV and then continued orally. Can you organize this tonight? Can you get a physiotherapist tomorrow? Can you review tomorrow? This will provide good palliation, but if the intent is to cure her then the risk is that this will be suboptimal treatment in view of her hypotension.
- To stay at home. Manage the pain with a small dose of morphine and review tomorrow. The intent here is to palliate symptoms but not prolong life.

Case history exercise: some thoughts on Mrs Pierce

To help us make the best decisions for Mrs Pierce we need to know as a much as possible about her.

- Before this pneumonia what was she able to do?
- What has the quality of her life been like in the past couple of months?

- Has she made any advance statements formally or had conversations with those close to her?
- Do her relatives know what her thoughts would be in her current situation?
- Does she appear distressed by physical things; pain, cough, breathing?
- Does she appear emotionally distressed; is she restless, clasping your hand, frowning? (She may of course not have the motor function to do any of these things.)

Remember that putting IV lines in and inserting nasogastric tubes have associated risks and discomfort. If the patient is dying, it can make the process clinical and not allow the relatives to be close. Drip stands and infusion lines can form an actual and indirect barrier around a patient. You must be sure that there are benefits to gain. You will need to keep this under review, as your approach may change over the next few days.

Unless she is able to cough, it is unlikely that her pneumonia will be cured by antibiotics alone. You need to make a decision about how 'active' you are going to be. Do you need further investigations to aid you in this (e.g. X-ray, blood gases, blood cultures)? Are they going to affect your management plan? Don't do them for the sake of it. Would ventilation be appropriate? You will need to discuss this with your senior doctor. The decision about her resuscitation status must also be documented.

Antibiotics may, however, reduce the quantity of sputum if this is distressing to her. If you decide to start them, you should review their benefit after 24 hours.

Mrs Pierce is unlikely to be distressed by thirst if good mouth care is undertaken by the nursing staff, in addition, fluid administration may cause pulmonary oedema. If your management plan is one of intensive treatment with a view to recovery, then fluids should be used with caution and their benefits and adverse effects be reviewed daily. If she gets worse, then you should plan to withdraw them.

Nutrition is not a clinical issue in the acute stage of her illness but the relatives may be concerned about it and you should discuss the fact that she does not need it immediately, that she is not hungry or suffering without it, and that it carries some risks while she is so ill. If she improves, this will of course need to be reviewed.

SUMMARY OF THE ETHICAL AND LEGAL CONSIDERATIONS:

What does she want?	Autonomy
Are you doing any good?	Beneficence
Are you doing any harm?	Non-maleficence
Is the intervention the best use of resources?	Justice
Are you obeying the law?	Legality

CHAPTER 5

Physical symptom control:
how to do it well

◆ Introduction *63*

◆ The principles of good symptom
  management *65*

◆ The management of pain *71*

◆ Nausea and vomiting *80*

◆ Intractable vomiting *81*

◆ Dyspnoea and cough *82*

◆ Constipation and diarrhoea *83*

◆ Symptom control in the last days of life *84*

◆ Case history exercise: some thoughts on the
  issues to anticipate and forward plan for
  Anna *86*

CHAPTER 5
Physical symptom control: how to do it well

Introduction

When asked about their experience in looking after patients in hospital some of your colleagues replied, 'Most SHOs/registrars are too busy passing examinations and moving on and most consultants are inadequately concerned in terminal care ... You are out on a limb and unsupported'.[1] The aim of this chapter is to help you feel equipped to be on the front line of managing symptoms and using controlled drugs, as you will be from day 1 as a junior doctor. Some of this will be about you learning how to approach clinical problems and some will be about gaining knowledge of what drugs and other therapies to use and how to prescribe them for best effect. However, some of it is about challenging yourself about your behaviour towards patients with pain, nausea, and distress of other sorts. In addition, providing care for patients in the very last stages of their lives has been found to be a challenge and a duty that many doctors shrink from.

> During ward rounds the four 'caring' consultants conducted comprehensive consultations and showed a holistic approach to care. Attention was paid to both the physical and psychosocial needs of patients ... The remaining 10 consultants concentrated on the patient's disease, the physical deterioration ... there was minimal or no personal contact with the patients ... When active medical intervention was scaled down and death was imminent they withdrew from the patient, either remaining at the foot of the bed or passing the patient's bed without comment or with a brief aside ... 'no change?' or 'still there?'
>
> Mills *et al.* (1994)[2]

How do you think that you will behave?

This chapter is not comprehensive in its coverage of symptoms and their management, and further sources of information are listed in Further reading at the end of the book. A wide range of drugs is available for symptom management and this can seem daunting. Familiarity and a good working knowledge of a relatively small group that you may need on a frequent basis is of prime importance, and these drugs are indicated in Appendix 2. Only morphine has been explored in any depth in this text and you should use other textbooks to familiarize yourself with the pharmacology of the others, including important side-effects, cautions and interactions, and methods of administration.

What physical symptoms do patients with advanced disease experience?

Several studies have shown a high prevalence of distressing physical problems experienced by patients with advanced disease (malignant and non-malignant) (Table 5.1). Pain is clearly a key symptom, but symptoms such as anorexia and fatigue are often paid little serious attention by professionals even though they have a very high prevalence and may be of great distress to patients and relatives.

LEARNING EXERCISE

What are the physical problems that you think patients experience? Elicit and list all the physical symptoms that the next three patients with advanced disease that you talk to have, and compare the list with Table 5.1. What additional problems do your patients have?

Improving outcomes for patients

Although we are well aware that physical symptoms in patients with advanced disease are common, many of these symptoms remain uncontrolled for patients.

Table 5.1 The probable prevalence of symptoms in advanced disease (derived from a variety of patient populations and study methodologies)

Symptom	Cancer (%)	Coronary heart disease (%)	Dementia (%)	AIDS (%)
Pain	60	60	65	60
Trouble breathing	40	50		10
Nausea or vomiting	40	45		20
Sleep disturbances	50			
Confusion	30	40	60	30
Fatigue/weakness	50		80	60
Depression	45	60	60	
Anorexia	60	40	60	40
Constipation	50	30		20
Incontinence	40		70	
Anxiety	40			

THINK POINT

Pain is uncontrolled in some 50% of patients with cancer in the UK.

If we were to use this as a performance indicator, we would be in the third division and being relegated. Why is this? Some symptoms are difficult to manage, but for the majority of patients a big difference can be made with low-tech, simple interventions requiring really quite a small amount of knowledge. Our experience has taught us that the key to achieving best symptom management is the application of principles and rules that underpin our care and incorporate factual knowledge and technical and communication skills.

Like becoming a good driver, you must have some *factual knowledge* about how the car works, what you must do *to make it go* and function at its *best performance*, and who to *ask for help* if it breaks down; but to get safely to where you want to go you must apply the principles and *rules of the highway code* (Figure 5.9).

The principles of good symptom management

Anticipation

It can often be anticipated that an individual patient may run in to specific problems, and in some instances you can prevent the predicted problem occur-

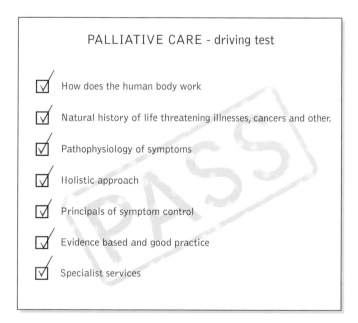

5.9 The keys to achieving good symptom control can be yours

> **Rule 1: Always think ahead**

ring. Thinking ahead gives you a better chance of nipping it in the bud before things require crisis management. Failure to anticipate problems and to set up appropriate management pathways (for instance, who should they call?) is a common source of dissatisfaction and preventable suffering for patients.

LEARNING EXERCISE

- What problems should you anticipate might occur when a patient starts taking codeine?
- What should you do to prevent them?

If you don't know the answers, the section of opioids later in this chapter should help you.

Understanding the natural history of the disease with specific reference to an individual patient, awareness of the patient's psychosocial circumstances, and identification of 'risk factors' allow forward planning of care by the healthcare team.

CASE HISTORY EXERCISE

Anna, a 45-year-old married woman with children aged 7 and 11, was recently found to have spinal metastases from her breast cancer.

Write short notes on the potential issues you should anticipate have a high risk of occurring for her in the future. Think about what, as her doctor, you will need to make sure is discussed and in place to prevent unnecessary suffering and crises, and to optimize symptom control.

(see our thoughts p. 86)

Evaluation and assessment

> **Rule 2: Always compile a differential diagnosis for the cause of symptom(s)**

An understanding of the pathophysiology and likely cause(s) of any particular problem is fundamental in selecting and directing appropriate investigations and treatment. When asked to see a patient to relieve distress, always, through careful history and examination, try to diagnose the cause of the symptom and decide whether it is possible and appropriate to remove the underlying cause or at least ameliorate it, in addition to providing concomitant symptomatic relief. For example:

LEARNING EXERCISE

Ask the next patient you see on regular opioids about his or her bowels. If constipated, ask them how this affects them. How embarrassing is it? Check the laxatives they are prescribed.

- Abdominal pain due to opioid-related constipation is better treated with suppositories or enemas than with opiates! (Have you seen this vicious circle in action? It is common.)
- Sedation for an agitated patient with urinary retention is not as helpful as catheterization.
- Antiemetics for the nausea of hypercalcaemia are important, but so may be lowering the serum calcium.

Be aware. Co-morbidity is common and should *always* be considered. For example, it is easy (and unfortunately common) to assume that pain in a patient with cancer is caused by the cancer. In one series almost a quarter of pains in patients with cancer were unrelated to the cancer or the cancer treatment.

> **Rule 3: Always consider the multidimensional (holistic) context of patients' symptoms**

The multidimensional nature of symptoms such as pain means that the use of drugs may be only part of a multiprofessional team strategy addressing physical, psychological, social, and spiritual distress. A patient's suffering always needs to be understood within its psychosocial context (see Chapter 3). Only by thinking holistically will we recognize those aspects of the patient's care that need approaches other than the use of drugs. For instance, the concept of total pain (see Chapter 3) acknowledges the importance of all of these dimensions of a person's suffering and that good pain relief is unlikely without attention to all of these areas.

Patients with chronic or advanced disease face many losses: loss of normality; loss of health; and potential loss of the future. Physical symptoms impose limitations on lifestyle. In addition, the symptom can be interpreted as an ever-present reminder of the underlying disease. NEVER underestimate the power of feelings in a patient's suffering.

> **Rule 4: Use treatments that address the pathophysiology of the symptom**

Deciding what treatment to use is based on evidence: evidence of the mechanism of the symptom and evidence of the treatment's efficacy and safety in that situation. Later in this chapter we give you some of the evidence. For example:

- 5-HT$_3$ antagonists are highly effective in the treatment of nausea of chemotherapy because of their effect on the chemoreceptor trigger zone and the gut. They are less effective than metoclopramide as an antiemetic for the nausea of gastric stasis.

KEY POINTS

To provide good symptom control you will have to THINK: what is causing this? UNDERSTAND: how does it cause that? KNOW: what is the best treatment for this cause?

- A distressing cough in a MND patient with aspiration pneumonia may be helped by antibiotics to reduce the generation of phlegm, physiotherapy to aid expectoration, and antitussive measures that include opioids that act on the brain-stem cough reflex (e.g. methadone and pholcodeine). Oropharyngeal local anaesthetic (spray or nebulized) may be helpful for patients in the last days of life to reduce the triggering of the cough reflex.

- A patient who is fearful of dying may be helped more by discussing and addressing specific fears rather than taking benzodiazepines.

Explanation and information

Rule 5: Management of a problem should always begin with sensitive explanation and discussion of the findings and diagnostic conclusions

Research and common sense tell us that most people wish to know what is going on with their bodies. What is happening and what to expect. This usually reduces the patient's anxieties, even if it confirms their worst suspicions. (A monster in the light is usually better faced than a monster unseen in the shadows.) A clear, sensitive explanation and discussion of the suggested treatments and follow-up plan is important for the patient to gain a sense of control and security and help them to share in decision making. Your skills in communication will be needed here (see Chapter 2).

Individualized treatment

The individual physical, social, and psychological circumstances of the patient and their views and wishes should be considered in planning care. This is why

THINK POINT

A patient asked me last week 'What sort of cancer have I got?' I wondered exactly what it was that she was wanting to know. 'Cancer of the cervix' I said. 'Yes, I know that, but what type is it?' she said. 'Do you mean you want to know how it looked under the microscope when they took the biopsy?' I asked cautiously. 'No, I mean is it the type that can be cured?' she said, rather exasperated with my obtuseness.

Rule 6: Treatments work best if they suit the individual patient

you need to share treatment options with patients. Don't come to them with a predetermined plan that they should comply with. When you get good at this you can even ask them first what they have in mind.

For example:

- The compression bandages for Mrs Stevens' lymphoedema treatment may be unused unless there is someone available to help her fit them daily.

- Mrs Jones may decline admission to get on top of her pain unless someone looks after her cat.

- Mr Singh may decline opioids because he wishes his mind to be clear on his journey towards death and the next life.

- Dr Peters had severe nausea with chemotherapy, pregnancy, and buprenorphine in the past. Starting an opioid for her pain control will need to take this into account and will require use of a prophylactic antiemetic.

> Having turned down the hideous jogging-suit provided by the hospital, I am now attired as I was in my student days. Like the bath, my old clothes could easily bring back poignant, painful memories. But I see in the clothes a symbol of continuing life. And proof that I still want to be myself. If I must drool, I may as well drool on cashmere.
>
> Jean-Dominique Bauby *The diving-bell and the butterfly*,
> HarperCollins Publishers Ltd.

Re-evaluation and supervision

Rule 7: Check to see that what you have done has worked

Symptoms can change frequently in advanced disease, especially when patients are frail. New problems can occur and established ones worsen. Proactive follow-up is vital.

If you have prescribed something to improve symptoms, check on its beneficial and adverse effects the next day. Getting on top of symptoms usually requires a few days of review and adjustment of medications or other measures. Sometimes more information from investigations is required. If things are not improving, asking a specialist palliative care team for additional advice is important. There

---

LEARNING EXERCISE

How does the hospital or primary-care team you are working in now seek specialist palliative care advice? Ask your house officer or GP trainer.

> **Rule 8: Seek specialist advice if problems are not improving**

should be specialist teams in the community and hospital settings. Often they are linked to Hospices (see Chapter 8).

When things are sorted, both the patient and healthcare team should know exactly who the patient or carer will contact if problems arise in future, especially out of normal working hours. Will there be a regular system for review? It is often useful to discuss with the patient and carer under what circumstances and where the patient should be admitted. Communicate your agreed plans clearly with all those involved, especially the patient's GP.

> **Rule 9: Plan follow-up and the safety net**

Attention to detail

The quality of palliative care is in the detail of care. For instance, it is vital to ensure that the patient not only has a prescription for the correct drug but also that he or she can obtain it from the pharmacy, has adequate supplies to cover a weekend, and understands how to adjust it if the problem worsens. Symptom control can be so finely balanced that the smallest of errors can make all the difference to the outcome.

> For half an hour the alarm on the machine regulating my feeding tube has been beeping out into the void. I cannot imagine anything so inane or nerve-racking as this piercing beep, beep, beep pecking away at the brain. To make matters worse, my sweat has unglued the tape that keeps my right eyelid closed, and the stuck-together lashes are tickling my pupil unbearably. To crown it all, the end of my urinary catheter has become detached and I am drenched.
>
> Jean Dominique Bauby *The diving-bell and the butterfly*
> HarperCollins Publishers Ltd.

Attention to detail is important in all of the aspects of symptom control outlined above. Without it resources and effort may be wasted and patients continue to suffer needlessly.

Continuing to care and providing continuity

It can be difficult for doctors to continue to make the time to care for patients in the very last stage of their lives. How do you prioritize this when patients who are acutely ill need the attention? Often, however, these patients are

> **Rule 10: Patients who are dying and their families need doctors to demonstrate that they continue to see their care, and them as people, as important**

LEARNING EXERCISE

For 1 day observe the care of a patient on your ward who your team are caring for as he or she dies. How much time did doctors and nurses spend with him or her and what did they do? Who spoke to the patient? What about? Can the patient manage to give him or herself a drink? Who helped with this? What three things, in your opinion, could easily be improved?

Mills *et al.*[2] give an example of this sort of observational study.

avoided because it is awkward and sad and we feel that there is nothing we can do. Helplessness is an uncomfortable feeling for a doctor. We like to be able to 'do' things.

However, it is important to remember the great value to the patient and their carers in continuing to stay involved, to acknowledge how difficult the situation is, not to abandon the patient because it is painful and distressing for the professional.

Continuity of care is also vital. No doctor can be available 24/7 but transfer of important information about the patient to doctors who take over the responsibility of care is vital. Some ways of doing this are:

- speaking to the doctor on call;
- clear notes to inform any healthcare professional;
- a summary letter held by the patient;
- patient-held records;
- providing contact details of the key healthcare team (see Rule 9).

The management of pain

The successful management of pain is one of the most satisfying experiences for a doctor. The GOOD NEWS is that in over 80% of patients with cancer-related pain it can be well controlled using low-cost, low-technology, straightforward methods. This probably holds true for most patients with pain related to non-malignant conditions. The BAD NEWS is that in general this is not achieved for patients. Key factors in this are the knowledge, skills, and attitudes of doctors. A salutory example of this, a letter from a staff nurse to the medical registrar on call, which explores some of the issues is reprinted as Fig. 5.1.

THINK POINT

Studies in the UK, USA, and Europe have shown that almost 50% of people with cancer-related pain receive inadequate relief.

Dear Doctor

He is dead now, so soon forgotten, but the fight and determination required to give this man a peaceful death will not be. All I asked for was 20 mg of diamorphine to be prescribed via continuous subcutaneous infusion over 24 hours to enable the patient who was terminally ill to remain pain free and peaceful while he bubbled and rattled, sweated and mottled his way out of this world. It was not much to ask.

A peaceful death is one to remember with gratitude by the relatives, giving a sense of relief and satisfaction to those nursing this decaying heap of humanity. The sight of a loved one in this terminal state is horrible, revolting, infinitely sad, but if their father, husband, or friend looks peaceful and pain free it is bearable.

So how was this request received by you the medical registrar? "He is not my patient." This was not true, you were on call for all the patients in the ward on that day. You refer to the drug list. "He is only on 5mg of diamorphine as required, let's increase the dose."

But this will only sedate the patient more heavily initially, and in time the effect of the analgesia will decrease, and once more distress and agitation will be evident. We can give him another injection and he will sink again into oblivion. But we nurses do not want to see pain and distress in this person who is so special to his friends and relatives gathered around his bed.

"Doctors should spend at least a month in a hospice as part of their training."

"Why are you asking for adequate pain relief at 4pm on a Sunday?" Yes, you really did say this. So once more you referred to the drug list. No, you did not look at the patient propped high on pillows, being turned every two hours, having his mouth cleaned, his airway aspirated, his eyes moistened, his necrosing flesh tended. No, you did not listen to and support the nurses who were tending this man for at least 15 minutes every two hours, who were supporting the relatives through many days of fading hope and increasing tiredness. Instead you raised

your voice, demonstrated your inexperience and lack of empathy and finally acquiesced, instructing your house officer to prescribe the requested drug before you stormed out of the ward stating you were not happy.

Well I was not happy. What if I was less experienced, had not seen how peaceful a death can be, had not the confidence to stand up to the doctor. This man would have suffered and his relatives would have long memories of distress and disappointment.

What is the solution? During medical school there must be modules relating to compassion and empathy. Medical students should understand that nurses tending the patient for hour after hour have greater insight into their needs than the doctors who may see them for five minutes a day. Doctors should spend at least a month in a hospice as part of their training before applying for a senior house officer or registrar job. And remember when a nurse asks for adequate pain relief it is for the patient's benefit so please listen to her with respect.

Yours sincerely
Staff Nurse Jones

Fig. 5.1 'Dear Doctor' (reprinted from the *British Medical Journal* 1996; 318; 888, with permission from the BMJ Publishing Group)

In general doctors are highly motivated to relieve suffering. So why then do we appear to fail our patients so often? How will you perform?

World Health Organization (WHO) analgesic ladder

Although the WHO analgesic ladder (Fig. 5.3)[3] was developed for use in cancer pain, a stepwise approach using a limited number of drugs is probably equally applicable to the management of chronic pain due to other causes, and has the potential to simplify prescribing. However, the use of strong opioids in non-malignant chronic pain is a controversial area and requires specialist advice and supervision.

The approach *combines* two modalities of pain relief:

● Non-opioid analgesics such as non-steroidal anti-inflammatory drugs (NSAIDs) or paracetamol reduce inflammation and/or prostaglandin synthesis and thereby reduce stimulation of nociceptors on peripheral nerves.

Managing cancer-related pain

Remember that pain is always a physical and emotional experience.
Lots of factors influence pain and how a patient copes with it. See the concept of total pain in Chapter 3.

Think—what is the cause of each of this patient's pains?	For each pain note: • characteristics • site • radiation • severity • onset	• exacerbating and relieving factors • effects of any drugs tried	What investigations may help? E.g. X-ray, bone scan
In the light of your assessment, what are the best drug and non-drug strategies for pain control?	Non-drug approaches include: • TENS • relaxation • hypnosis	• acupuncture • radiotherapy • surgery	Pattern recognition *(see table below)*	The WHO analgesic ladder (see Fig. 5.3)
Use a multi-professional, holistic, team approach	Ask the patient or nurse to use a pain chart to assess progress	Physio- and occupational therapists are essential for managing incident pain	Plan when and who will make sure there is satisfactory progress
Explain to patient and family and review the patient early	What does this pain mean to the patient?	Many people feel that severe pain is inevitable in cancer, and this may lead to fear, suffering, and reluctance to ask for help. Pain may be erroneously interpreted by patients as an indication of progression of their cancer and therefore a signal of their approaching death

Recognize patterns of pain

Type of pain	Key features	Response to opioids	Comments
Soft tissue	Localized ache throbbing, gnawing	Good	>80% pain control easily achievable by non-opioid ± opioid
Visceral	Poorly localized deep ache. Pain may be referred to specific sites	Good	>80% pain control easily achievable by non-opioid ± opioid
Bone	Well localized aching pain, local tenderness	Variable	Non-steroid anti-inflammatory drugs (NSAIDs) + radiotherapy are important treatment options
Neuropathic (see text)	Difficult to describe; dysaesthesia; associated motor/sensory loss; pain distributed in specific dermatomal, radicular, or nerve territory	Often poor	Adjuvant treatments usually needed; early referral for specialist advice improves outcome
Incident pain	Occurs episodically: on movement, weight bearing, change of dressing, etc.	Moderate	Find ways to avoid provocation. Consider: • extra analgesics before predictable provocation • gaseous nitrous oxide • spinal routes of analgesia • orthopaedic interventions for spinal stabilization and strengthening weight-bearing bones

> **If you need any help with a patient you can contact the palliative care team in hospital or community**

Fig. 5.2 A guide to the successful management of cancer-related pain

WHO Analgesic ladder

By the clock

Chronic pain such as cancer pain is continuous—use regular analgesia at appropriate dose intervals, not P.R.N. Using regular analgesia to prevent reoccurrence of pain will lead to better pain control with lower daily doses of analgesia and probably fewer side-effects. Just as importantly, this will also gain patients' confidence in your ability to get their pain under control

By the mouth

The oral route is preferred for all steps of the analgesic 'ladder'. The oral route gives patients more control and is less disruptive. It is effective patient-controlled analgesia unless medicines are not able to be ingested or absorbed

Start at the first step on the ladder and move upwards to titrate analgesia to control pain

Adjuvant analgesics may be helpful at any stage of the ladder (see text and Fig. 5.2)

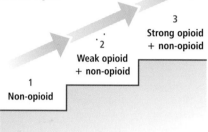

1
Non-opioid

2
Weak opioid + non-opioid

3
Strong opioid + non-opioid

Non-opioid analgesics

Paracetamol is a good analgesic and most patients experience few side effects. However the maximum dose is restricted by hepatotoxicity. It may be sufficient analgesia for some patients. More usually it is part of the analgesic regime and is combined with opioids.

NSAIDs have more side effects than paracetamol but are excellent anti-inflammatory analgesics. Common and important side-effects are ulceration of the upper GI tract with pain, nausea, bleeding, and renal function impairment

Opioid analgesics

See text

Breakthrough pain

Transitory exacerbations of pain are common and sometimes predictable (see incident pain in Fig. 5.2). Patients should *always* have access to extra analgesia for these episodes (e.g. morphine ⅙th daily dose)

Reduce side-effects

Side-effects of opioids (strong and weak): approximate incidence with appropriate use in cancer pain treatment

Constipation	90%
Nausea	30%
Vomiting	10%
Dry mouth	50%
Drowsiness	10%
Confusion	10%
Reduced respiratory rate	<1%
Addiction	<1%

Fig. 5.3 The WHO analgesic ladder for cancer pain management

- Opioids reduce transmission of nociceptive stimuli to the conscious brain through inhibition at opioid receptors in the brain-stem, spinal cord, and perhaps in peripheral nerves.

However, as indicated in the table in Fig. 5.2 a variable response to opioids should be anticipated and in some patients the addition of adjuvant analgesic agents is important in achieving pain control.

Weak opioid analgesics

Codeine, dextroproxyphene, and dihydrocodeine are used in combination with a non-opioid analgesic such as paracetamol, at the second step of the ladder. Tablets containing a combination of weak opioids and paracetamol are readily available. There is a 'ceiling' to the effect of weak opioids (usually two tablets four times daily) and if regular, maximum doses do not achieve adequate analgesia, then you should take a step up the ladder, i.e. the weak opioid should be replaced with strong opioid, usually morphine. There is no advantage in changing to an alternative opioid for mild to moderate pain.

Strong opioid analgesics

> If judiciously and freely administered it [opium] is equal to most of the emergencies in the way of pain, that we are likely to meet with in the dying, whereas timidly and inadequately used, the sufferer is deprived of the relief which it alone is capable of affording.
>
> William Munk, 1887 (famous Victorian physician who wrote the first textbook on caring for the dying patient)

In the UK morphine, derived from opium, remains the strong opioid of first choice. When using morphine and other strong opioids the following points should be remembered:

- Explain the drug to the patient and their carer. Anticipate that they may have significant concerns, which need to be addressed.

- Prevention of side-effects: use a prophylactic stimulant laxative such as senna or dantron; consider an antiemetic.

LEARNING EXERCISE What worries people about using morphine?

- Write a list of 10 things you anticipate that your patients may be worried about when you suggest they start morphine.
- Now think how you will alleviate their worries.
- Check these thoughts out with the next patient you see who is on, or about to start, morphine for chronic pain.
- What might worry *you*? How might you put patients at risk and how will you ensure good risk management? There are risks both in prescribing too little and too much morphine. Read on to reduce your worries about this and increase your competence.

Using morphine: Step 1, gain control of pain

- Titrate the dose needed for pain relief by using immediate-release morphine (elixir or tablets). The starting dose for those patients that have been on regular weaker opioids is 10 mg 4 hourly (i.e. 6 times daily). In the elderly or those with renal

KEY POINTS

Make sure you are competent in the use of opioids before you qualify.

impairment, smaller doses (2.5–5 mg) and closer monitoring are required.

- Ensure that patients have access to the same dose of morphine for break-through pain on an as-required (p. r. n.) basis.
- Reassess pain control daily.
- Titrate the dose to achieve pain relief by a 30–50% increment in dose every 2–3 days, or sooner if necessary.
- Remember to increase the p. r. n. dose for breakthrough pain.
- Doubling the dose at bedtime may avoid the need for an early morning dose.
- A 'log' of treatment and its effect is help-ful in titration if the patient is at home.
- If your patient's pain does not improve within 3 days, or there are severe side-effects, seek specialist help.

> **KEY POINTS**
>
> - Two-thirds of patients need up to 200 mg morphine per day.
> - One-third of patients may need higher doses, up to 1200 mg morphine per day, and occasionally more.

Using morphine: Step 2, maintenance of pain control

Once pain is controlled consider, with the patient:

- a longer-acting preparation (12 hourly or 24 hourly) equivalent to the total daily dose of morphine;
- an alternative mode of delivery (e.g. fentanyl patch).

In addition, persistent morphine-related side-effects may be less with an alter-native strong opioid (seek specialist advice).

A patient should never be prescribed more than one modified release opioid at a time, and all patients on long-acting opioid preparations require a immediate-release, short-acting opioid to be available for episodes of break-through pain. This is usually morphine and the dose should be equivalent to one-sixth of the total daily dose.

Converting between strong opioids

This may be useful for patients who:

- require non-oral opioids (transdermal or subcutaneous infusion);
- have intolerable opioid-related side-effects, which may be drug specific;
- use high doses of opioids with apparent tolerance to its analgesic effects.

Except for coversion to diamorphine (shown in Table 5.2) this will usually require specialist advice.

Table 5.2 Conversion between oral morphine and subcutaneous (SC) diamorphine (3 mg oral morphine = 1 mg SC diamorphine)

Opioid and route	Equivalent dose		
Oral morphine (mg/24 h)	90	180	240
SC diamorphine for infusion (mg/24 h)	30	60	80
SC diamorphine for breakthrough pain (mg)	5	10	15

Neuropathic pain and the use of adjuvant analgesics

Pain that arises because of damage to the nervous system is particularly unpleasant, difficult for patients to describe, and problematic to manage. Specialist advice is often required and you should seek this early for any patient you think has neuropathic pain, since it seems that the longer it is left untreated the harder it is to resolve.

Patients experience a variety of abnormal sensations in neuropathic pain, which have specific terminologies. Differentiating these may give guidance to pathophysiology of the nerve damage and the best modality of treatment. Pain in an area of numbness is a pathognomonic indicator of neuropathic pain.

Nervous tissue may be damaged by a variety of insults, for example:

- infarction, e.g. central post-stroke pain;

- infection, e.g. HIV-related neuropathy;

- drugs, e.g. post-chemotherapy neuropathy;

- trauma, e.g. radiculopathy associated with spinal cord compression.

The management of such pains is largely a postgraduate subject, but you should be aware that the general approach is to employ the WHO analgesic ladder and that 'adjuvant' analgesics are frequently required.

An adjuvant analgesic is a drug that is not generally classified as an analgesic but has a pain-relieving effect in particular circumstances. The evidence base

---

Abnormal sensations in neuropathic pain

Dysaesthesia: spontaneous and evoked abnormal sensation.
Hyperaesthesia: an increased non-painful sensitivity to non-painful stimulation, e.g. touch.
Hyperalgesia: increased response (intensity and duration) to a stimulus that is normally painful.
Allodynia: pain caused by a stimulus that is not normally painful.
Hyperpathia: explosive and often prolonged painful response to a non-painful stimulus.

for the use of such drugs is very slim, and trials have been undertaken mostly in patients with trigeminal neuralgia, post-herpetic neuralgia, and diabetic neuropathy. Table 5.3 outlines the use of the key first-line adjuvant analgesic drugs. For many patients, unresolvable side-effects limit the dose of the drug, especially for patients who are also on opioids.

Table 5.3 Adjuvant analgesics for neuropathic pain

Drug group	Probable main mechanism of action	Typical regime
Tricyclic antidepressants	Enhance central inhibition by increase in synaptic serotonin	Amitriptyline 10–25 mg at night increased slowly to a maximum of 150 mg/24 h
Anticonvulsants	Decrease neuronal excitability	Carbamazepine 200 mg twice a day. Increase slowly to a maximum of 1.5 g/24 h
		Gabapentin 100–300 mg at night. Increase slowly to a maximum of 600 mg three times daily
Steroids	Reduce perineural oedema	Dexamethasone 6 mg in the morning. Higher dose (16 mg) may be useful, e.g. in spinal cord compression

Nausea and vomiting

Think—why is this patient vomiting?	Only by making a reasoned judgement as to the cause of a patient's vomiting do you stand a chance of controlling this common symptom. Consider: • the disease process itself • complications of the disease process • side-effects of drugs • previous drugs used • complications of other treatments • psychosocial factors • the characteristics of the nausea and vomiting

In the light of your assessment; reverse the reversible, use the most appropriate non-drug and drug methods to control it (see table)

Classifications	Causes*	Characteristics	First-line drugs	Second-line drugs
Upper GI stasis/outflow obstruction	• tumour • anticholinergic drugs • hepatomegaly	• epigastric discomfort • worse on eating • eased by vomiting • variable nausea	metoclopramide 10–20 mg TDS oral 30–60 mg/24 h SC	domperidone 10–20 mg TDS oral 30–60 mg/24 h SC
Chemically induced	• drugs • metabolic • toxic	• constant nausea • variable vomiting	haloperidol 1.5–5 mg oral 1.5–5 mg/24 h SC	metoclopromide 10–20 mg t.d.s. oral 30–60 mg/24 h SC
Constipation	• drugs • because of cancer • immobility	• nausea and faeculant vomiting • associated with constipation	stimulant and softener laxative (e.g. co-danthramer 10 ml at night)	laxative and glycerine or bisacodyl suppositories
Raised intracranial pressure	• cerebral mets • cerebral haemorrhage	• nausea worse in the morning • projectile vomiting • worse on head movement	trial of steroids Dexamethasone 8–16 mg/24 h oral/SC/IM/IV	Cyclizine 25–50 mg t.d.s. oral 100–150 mg/24 h
Intestinal obstruction	• malignant • non malignant	• vomiting with abdominal pain, distension and constipation	hyoscine butylbromide 60–200 mg/24 h SC	trial of octreotide 200 μg up to 600 μg/24 h SC
Anxiety	• any cause	• symptoms worse when anxious	Diazepam 2–5 mg t.d.s.	
Unknown cause	If you cannot discern a reason for your patient's nausea and vomiting		Cyclizine 25–50 mg t.d.s. oral 100–150 mg/24 h SC	

* Remember: **many causes can be treated without long-term anti-emetics** (e.g. stopping causative drugs, treating constipation, reversing metabolic disturbance, treating infection, surgical treatment, etc.)

t.d.s., three times daily; SC, subcutaneously; IM, intramuscularly; IV, intravenously.

If prescribing an anti-emetic, then must have a very good reason to use oral route

Explain to patient and family and review the patient early

If you need any help with a patient you can contact the palliative care team in hospital or community

Intractable vomiting

Although the principles described opposite will be successful in many cases there are some cases where control is harder to achieve. Then you may need to prescribe more than one anti-emetic, or use use different drugs. When doing this it helps if you understand the neurophysiology, so that you don't prescribe inappropriately.

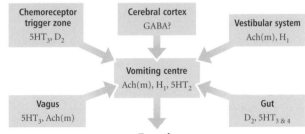

Chemoreceptor trigger zone	Cerebral cortex	Vestibular system
$5HT_3, D_2$	GABA?	$Ach(m), H_1$

Vomiting centre
$Ach(m), H_1, 5HT_2$

Vagus	Gut
$5HT_3, Ach(m)$	$D_2, 5HT_{3 \& 4}$

Emesis

Receptor site affinities of selected anti-emetics

Drug name	D_2	H_1	Ach(m)	$5HT_2$	$5HT_3$	$5HT_4$	GABA
Metachlopromide	●●	–	–	–	(●)	●●	–
Domperidone	●●	–	–	–	–	–	–
Ondansetron	–	–	–	–	●●●	–	–
Cyclizine	–	●●	●●	–	–	–	–
Hyoscine	–	–	●●●	–	–	–	–
Haloperidol	●●●	–	–	–	–	–	–
Prochlorperazine	●●	●	–	–	–	–	–
Levomepromazine	●●	●●	●●	●●●	–	–	–
Diazepam	–	–	–	–	–	–	●●

Key

D_2	Dopamine type 2 receptors
H_1	Histamine type 1 receptors
Ach(m)	Muscarinic cholinergic
$5HT_{2,3,4}$	Serotonin type 2, 3 and 4
GABA	Gamma-amino-butyric acid
–	no affinity
●	slight affinity
●●	moderate affinity
●●●	marked affinity

Useful points:

- Don't use the IM route if you can help it—it's painful!
- Ensure any anti-emetic used is given regularly: anti-emetics as required are never going to control regular nausea and vomiting
- Use any anti-emetic to maximum dosage before swapping
- If first drug is unsuccessful, try one from a different group
- Don't use two drugs from the same group on the same patient
- Haloperidol and Cyclizine are often a successful combination
- Anti-cholinergic drugs have predictable side effects and can antagonise metochlopromide and other prokinetic drugs
- Consider non-drug methods (e.g. acupuncture, ginger, relaxation, hypnotherapy, control malodour, avoid certain foods, small meals)
- Pain and coughing can cause vomiting
- For intractable vomiting it may be worth trying:
  - Levomepromazine 6.25–50 mg OD orally or 6.25–12.5 mg/24 h SC
  - three day trial of dexamethasone 4–20 mg/24 h
  - three day trial of ondansetron 8 mg BD or TDS

> If you need any help with a patient you can contact the palliative care team in hospital or community

Dyspnoea and cough

| Think—why is the patient short of breath? | There is often more than one cause for dyspnoea. **Common causes** to consider are:

• Anxiety
• Lung cancer (primary or secondary)
  • Obstruction of bronchus
  • Effusion
• Anaemia
• Concurrent lung disease
• Loss of respiratory muscle
• Splinting of diaphragm
• Pulmonary embolus

If possible watch the patient walk: it tells you a lot. | **When to order tests?**
This can be tricky. Chest X-ray, full blood count, and sputum microbiology may be useful diagnostically. |

In the light of your assessment; reverse the reversible, use the most appropriate non-drug and drug methods to control it (see table) Listening, understanding and reassuring are vitally important

Specific treatment for specific causes

Anxiety	General measures and diazepam (see below)
Lung cancer	• Speak to oncologist about radiotherapy, chemotherapy • Consider pleural drainage if effusion present
Anaemia	Consider transfusion. Always check; did they improve and for how long?
Concurrent lung disease	Antibiotics (infection), Bronchodilators (COPD/asthma), diuretics (CCF), etc.
Loss of respiratory muscle	General measures (see below)
Splinting of diaphragm	Drain ascites if present, otherwise general measures and non-specific drug options (see below)
Pulmonary embolus	Anticoagulation not always necessary. Analgesia and general measures

Non-specific treatment for general symptom control

General measures; can be considered in all patients whatever the cause	• Give the patient time and reassurance • Relaxation • Breathing techniques • Open window or fan • Positioning for maximal breathing • Consider physio or occupational therapy referral
Non-specific drug options	• Diazepam 2–5 mg TDS, reduced to once a day when stable • Morphine 2.5 mg every 4 hours if not on opioids, titrating up according to response. If on opioids, make a 30–50% increase in dose. • Oxygen. In the hypoxic (PaO_2 <9)

What about cough?

• Treat the cause; cancer, antibiotics, diuretics, bronchodilators
• Nebulized saline if tenacious sputum
• Simple linctus 5 ml, 3–4 times a day
• Codeine linctus 5–10 ml, 3–4 times a day

COPD, chronic obstructive pulmonary disease; CCF, congestive cardiac failure.

Involve the patient and key individuals in all stages and agree follow-up

---

If you need any help with a patient you can contact the palliative care team in hospital or community

Constipation and diarrhoea

Constipation

Remember this is a common problem so always ask about it.
Common causes are:

* drugs, especially opioids
* poor oral intake
* immobility
* gut cancers
* co-morbidity (e.g. diverticular disease)

Think—why has this patient got constipation or diarrhoea?

Diarrhoea

Common causes to think about are:

* over use of laxatives
* other drugs (e.g. antibiotics)
* constipation with overflow
* side-effect of pelvic radiotherapy
* malabsorption from bowel resections or pancreatic malfunction
* tumour invasion of gut wall
* infection
* fistula
* co-morbidity

---

* reverse the cause if possible
* always prescribe a laxative with an opioid
* titrate the dose up to get a result
* think carefully and consider patient's embarrassment

Laxatives

* use a stimulant and softener combined (e.g. co-danthrusate 2 capsules or 10 ml at night. Latency of 6–12 hours)

Rectal treatments
(may or may not be needed)

* *hard faeces:* soften with glycerine suppositories
* *soft faeces:* stimulate with bisacodyl suppositories
* *empty rectum:* consider obstruction or phosphate enema

In the light of your assessment, what are the best strategies for good symptom control?

Cause	Treatment
laxatives, antibiotics, antacids, chemotherapy	stop drugs if possible
constipation with overflow	laxatives and suppositories/ enemas
malabsorption	pancreatic supplements, bilary stenting
tumour invasion of gut wall	palliative radiotherapy or chemotherapy
infection	treatment guided by culture and sensitivity
co-morbidity	treat according to condition
cause unknown or specific treatment ineffective	Loperamide up to 16 mg daily Codeine 10–60 mg daily Octreotide SC (seek specialist advice)

Liaise closely with rest of team when making decision, and fully support good nursing care. Involve the patient and their carers as much as possible in the decision making and be clear about follow-up

Remember:
Oral rehydration, low-fibre diet and the importance of good nursing care

---

If you need any help with a patient you can contact the palliative care team in hospital or community

Symptom control in the last days of life

Dying people require a truly holostic approach to their care. Many physical problems arise and comfort is essential, but so too is consideration of place of care, their need for religious ritual or prayer, and support for their relatives. Attention to detail and continued involvement of the clinical team are paramount. The non-physical aspects of care have been discussed in other chapters. You should take the following approach:

Is the patient dying?	Patients who are dying may often be:	

Patients who are dying may often be:

- profoundly weak
- gaunt
- drowsy
- disorientated

- having difficulty taking things orally
- breathing in abnormal patterns

- unable to concentrate
- reducing peripheral perfusion with skin colour and temperature changes

---

Is he/she comfortable?

What do I need to decide?

What should I anticipate?

General considerations

Review drip, drugs, and other interventions

Can you stop:

- drugs
- IV fluids
- blood tests
- routine observations?

It is likely that many are not helpful at this stage.

Route of drug administration

- Use syringe driver for SC medications (see Chapter 6).
- Use NSAID per rectum (PR) for stiffness and bone pain.

Common symptoms

Extreme fatigue

Patients need anyone and everyone to help with a drink or repositioning a pillow

Excess respiratory secretions

- optimize the patient's position in bed
- use suction
- use an anticholinergic agent:
  Hyoscine butylbromide SC 20 mg stat: 60–120 mg/24 h
  Hyoscine hydrobromide SC 200 μg stat: 600–1200 μg/24 h

Mouth care

- Hourly nursing attention
- Vaseline to lips

Terminal restlessness and agitation

The reasons may be multiple, E.g. hypotension, hypoxia, biochemical abnormalities.

Most patients are very frightened.

It is very distressing to carers.

It is perhaps the most difficult symptom to manage at home.

- Exclude an obvious cause for distress (e.g. full bladder, wet bed.)
- Reassure the patient and talk to the family about what is happening.
- Try and establish a quiet, low-stimulation environment for the patient.

Medication, usually parenteral, may be needed if the patient is a danger to him/herself or clearly very distressed:

Where delirium and psychotic features are predominant:
haloperidol SC 5 mg stat and 5–10 mg/24 h
or
levomepromazine SC 12.5–25 mg stat or 12.5–100 mg/24 h

Where anguish and anxiety are predominant:
midazolam SC 2–10 mg then 5–30 mg/24 h
or
diazepam 5–10 mg PR

Have I talked to the patient and the relatives?
See Chapters 2, 3 and 4

If you need any help with a patient you can contact the palliative care team in hospital or community

Case history exercise: some thoughts on the issues to anticipate and forward plan for Anna

The common issues that may arise for Anna are:

- Pain: may need NSAIDs, opioid, and radiotherapy.
- Spinal cord compression (see below): neurological examination if she says she is unsteady or 'numb'.
- Anxiety about her young children: she may need help, practically and in telling the children.
- Work: she may need financial, benefit, and employment advice.
- Hypercalcaemia: check blood if nauseated or confused.

It is particularly important that you are competent in assessing, diagnosing, and managing potential spinal cord compression. If you suspect spinal cord compression, then you must seek urgent oncological assessment. For further information see *Oncology: An Oxford Core text*, Spence and Johnston (2001) and *Handbook of Palliative Care*, Faull *et al*. (1998).

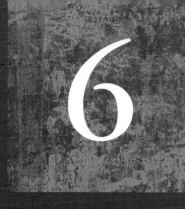

6

CHAPTER 6

*The syringe driver: a useful
way to deliver drugs*

- Introduction *89*

- Graseby MS 16 and MS 26 syringe
  drivers *90*

- Frequently asked questions *91*

- Problem preventing and solving *98*

- Case history exercise: some thoughts on the
  plan of management for Jane *99*

CHAPTER 6

The syringe driver: a useful way to deliver drugs

Introduction

It is quite common that patients with advanced illness cannot take their medications orally. This is always a good time to review the necessity to continue all drugs, many of which can be stopped at this time. However, maintaining good symptom management may require established medications (such as analgesics) to continue, or the addition of other medicines. An alternative to the oral route of drug delivery is needed. Some drugs can be given rectally (PR) but many require, or the patient would prefer, parenteral administration. The subcutaneous (SC) route is less painful than intramuscular (IM) and much more convenient than intravenous (IV). Many drugs can be delivered SC, but some must be given IM or IV or an alternative drug substituted.

Drugs used for symptom management which can *not* be given SC	
Chlorpromazine	Phenytoin
Prochlorperazine	Diazepam

Drugs used for symptom management which could be given PR	
Diazepam	Prochlorperazine
Diclofenac	Domperidone
Naproxen	Morphine

In palliative care, using a small, battery-operated, portable infusion pump, usually referred to as a 'syringe driver' has become a firmly established method of administering subcutaneous infusions of analgesic, anti-emetic, sedative, and anticholinergic drugs. For some patients this is an interim measure while problems such as vomiting are controlled, for others it is a way of delivering medicines to ensure comfort in the last days of their life.

Indications for using a syringe driver

◆ Persistent nausea

◆ Vomiting

◆ Difficulty swallowing

◆ Poor gastrointestinal absorption

◆ Intestinal obstruction

◆ Profound weakness

◆ Comatose patient

CASE HISTORY EXERCISE

Jane has advanced intra-abdominal ovarian cancer. She has been admitted to the surgical ward today with vomiting for 2 days, which has become faeculent. She has been constipated for 2 weeks. She is very frail. She has been taking sustained release morphine 40 mg 12 hourly and because she hasn't kept this down she is now in considerable pain. She is nauseated but has little colic. Her husband tells you that they know no surgery will be possible and that they would, most of all, like to be at home if only she can be more comfortable.

As Jane's doctor what will you need to know to provide Jane with the best care? (see our thoughts p. 99)

This chapter will discuss the practicalities of both the use of the syringe driver and the administration of drugs by subcutaneous infusion.

Graseby MS 16 and MS 26 syringe drivers

Two of the most commonly used syringe drivers are the Graseby MS 16 (blue), with a rate setting at mm/h, and the Graseby MS 26 (green), with a rate setting at mm/24 h (Fig. 6.1).

Syringe drivers allow patients to be as ambulant as possible and avoid the necessity for repeated injections (important in frail, cachectic patients). They can be used in the hospital and at home. Some patients, however, find the syringe driver obtrusive and disconcerting.

Since it is frequently used to deliver medications in the last days of life it is sometimes seen by both patients and staff as synonymous with a last rite. This is a mistake, and since staff, patients, and families may make wrong-

KEY POINTS

◆ Not everyone who is dying needs a syringe driver.

◆ Not everyone with a syringe driver is dying.

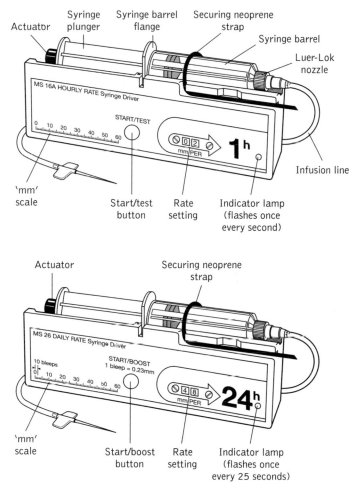

Fig. 6.1 The two syringe drivers most commonly used to deliver SC infusions of drugs for symptom control

ful assumptions about the use of syringe drivers for delivery of medications at earlier stages in advanced disease, it is always important to explain the rationale for the use of the syringe driver and the overall aims of care. Invite questions, acknowledge anxieties, and reassure where appropriate.

Frequently asked Questions

How do you set up a syringe driver?

This is usually done by nurses, but all doctors should also be competent in order to ensure safe prescribing and administering of medicines.

Setting up a syringe driver

You will need:

- syringe driver
- battery
- Luer-Lok syringe (usually 10 ml but 20 ml may be used)
- infusion or (giving) set (choose the smallest volume)
- fine-gauge butterfly needle (23G or 25G)
- clear adhesive dressing (e.g. Opsite[R])
- diluent (usually water for injection)
- medication as prescribed.

Preparing the infusion

1. Draw back the plunger on the empty syringe until the volume of air measures 48 mm in length (measure on a ruler or on the scale on the syringe driver).

2. Note the air volume that measures 48 mm in length.

3. Dissolve powdered drugs to be used with sterile water for injection.

4. Draw up drugs into the syringe and dilute, with sterile water for injection, to the volume noted in 2 above.

5. Invert the syringe several times to ensure good mixing.

6. If you are initiating treatment, connect the infusion (giving) set to the Luer-Lok and prime the infusion line (i.e. fill the whole giving set to needle tip).

7. Label the syringe clearly with the patient's name and infusion contents

Preparing the syringe driver

8. Insert battery; alarm will sound for a few seconds.

9. Press start/boost button. The motor will run for a short while safety circuits are checked.

10. Release start button.

11. Set the rate of delivery. Usually medicines are delivered over 24 h. The rate of delivery is calculated as :

$$\frac{\text{length of volume (e.g. 48 mm)}}{\text{delivery time} \quad 24\,\text{h}}$$

KEY POINT

BE AWARE
Check the rate setting *very carefully* as they are very different for the two types of syringe driver

With 48 mm of infusion: the MS 16 is set at 02 mm/h
the MS 26 is set at 48 mm/24 hr

Attach the loaded syringe to syringe driver

The syringe sits on top of the driver in a shallow v-shaped recess: fit the flange of the barrel into the slot provided.

12. Secure in position with the neoprene strap.

13. Press the white release button to slide the actuator assembly up to the plunger, and clamp in place.

Commencing the infusion

14. Insert fine-gauge butterfly or giving set into the skin at an angle of 45 degrees to the skin.

15. Start the driver by pressing the start button; the light will flash every 20–25 seconds.

16. Protect the mixture from light by using a holster or covering.

17. If this is the initiation of treatment or a newly primed giving set, note that the infusion will go through in less than 24 h because of the 'dead space' volume of the giving set (e.g. if the dead space volume is 1 ml and the 48 mm 'volume' is 9 ml, then the syringe will be empty in 21 h 20 min.) Incorporate this in the plan for recharging the infusion.

SC infusion sites

Suitable subcutaneous infusion sites:

- anterior chest wall
- upper arms
- abdominal wall.

Sites to avoid:

- lymphoedematous limb
- Areas of inflammation
- broken skin.

LEARNING EXERCISE

Ask the nursing staff on your ward if you can watch them set up the next syringe driver.

Why is the infusion rate in mm not ml?

The Graseby pumps are designed and calibrated to move the syringe plunger by a set length (mm) in a set time (h). Movement of the syringe plunger will deliver a variable volume of syringe contents, dependant on the bore of the syringe. The syringe bore varies both with the syringe volume (i.e. 20 ml syringes are wider than 10 ml syringes) and with manufacturer (i.e. not all 10 ml syringes are the same width).

What is of prime importance when you prescribe the infusion is not the volume but the *length* of the infusion in the syringe. This is very different from other sorts of pumps we may use to deliver larger volumes of infusions. To deliver drugs by infusion over 24 h a length of 48 mm is usually prescribed. It just makes the maths easy when setting the rate of mm/h (i.e. 48 is divisible by 24).

Illustrative example

Two syringes both contain 60 mg of diamorphine. Syringe A is a 10 ml and syringe B is a 20 ml syringe. The diamorphine has been mixed with water for injection and both syringes have been filled to a volume measuring 48 mm in length. For syringe A, 48 mm length is 9.2 ml and for syringe B 48 mm length is 16.4 ml You want both syringes to deliver their infusion over 24 h and have set the two MS16 drivers to 02 mm/h.

What volume is being delivered each hour by the two syringes?

Syringe A:
Movement of the plunger by 2 mm delivers 9.2/48 × 2 ml of infusion = 0.38ml.

Syringe B:
Movement of the plunger by 2 mm delivers 16.4/48 × 2 ml of infusion = 0.68 ml.

How long does it take for the infusion to begin working?

At least 4 hours. So if the patient needs immediate interventions (e.g. for pain) they will require a stat (bolus) dose of relevant drugs at the same time as commencing the subcutaneous continuous infusion.

What is the boost button for?

The boost button on the MS 26 is also the start button and is generally **only used to start the infusion.** Pressing the boost button during the infusion moves the syringe plunger by 0.23 mm. This delivers a *very* small amount of

the infusion, far from sufficient to relieve breakthrough pain, for example, for which the equivalent of a 4-hourly dose of opioid is recommended. In addition, all the drugs in the infusion are 'boosted', not just the one desired. For the purposes of symptom management the boost button is therefore a misnomer and if patients require extra medication, this should be delivered by an additional SC injection.

What drugs can you deliver subcutaneously?

Although subcutaneous administration of the drugs indicated in Table 6.1 is common and accepted good practice in palliative care, the use of this route lies outside the product licence for most of these preparations. Only levomepromazine is licensed for subcutaneous use. This does not preclude their use in this way, but this is a particular clinical governance issue (see also Chapter 7).

What is the best opioid to use and how do I calculate the dose?

Diamorphine is the opioid of choice for injection because of its high solubility.

3 mg oral morphine =
1 mg diamorphine injection

To convert from oral morphine to subcutaneous diamorphine, divide the total 24 h morphine dose by 3 to obtain the total 24 h diamorphine dose.

Use opioid conversion tables and seek specialist pharmacy or palliative care advice when converting from opioids other than morphine.

What drugs can you mix in the same syringe?

Table 6.2 indicates the compatibility of two drug combinations. Where it is indicated that caution is required at higher concentrations, specialist pharmaceutical advice should be sought. In general, the combination of more than two drugs should be avoided. Exceptions for common clinical practice, for doses of diamorphine up to 50 mg/ml, are:

- diamorphine + midazolam + hyoscine hydrobromide;
- diamorphine + midazolam + haloperidol;
- diamorphine + levomepromazine + hyoscine hydrobromide.

What should I do if the dose of a drug needs to be changed?

Reviewing the patient's needs daily will often lead you to make changes to the pre-

Don't alter the rate; use a newly made up syringe with the new prescription

Table 6.1 Medicines commonly used for symptom management

Medication	Indication	S.C. Starting dose/24 h & (Range)
Opioid Diamorphine	Pain	• 1/3 total dose of oral morphine. • 10–20 mg (starting dose if not already taking opioids) • Increasing as necessary by 30–50% increments
	Dyspnoea	
Antiemetic		
Metoclopramide	Impaired gastric emptying	30 mg (30–60 mg)
Haloperidol	) Drug induced and) metabolic causes of) nausea	5 mg (2.5–10 mg)
Cyclizine	) Intestinal obstruction	150 mg (50–150 mg)
Sedative & Antiemetic		
levomepromazine	Nausea	12.5 mg (2.5–25 mg)
	Sedation, confusion, agitation, terminal restlessness	25 mg (12.5–100 mg)
Sedative		
Midazolam	Terminal restlessness Myoclonic jerking Anticonvulsant	10–30 mg (range 10–90 mg)
Anticholinergic		
Hyoscine Hydrobromide (also antiemetic)	Terminal bronchial secretions	0.6 mg (0.6–2.4 mg)
	Severe colic	
Hyoscine Butylbromide	Intestinal obstruction	60-mg (60–180 mg)
Steroid		
Dexamethasone	Reduction in peritumour oedema	4 mg (2–16 mg)

Table 6.2 The compatibility of drugs combined in a syringe for SC infusion

	Diamorphine	Metoclopramide	Haloperidol	Cyclizine	Levomepromazine	Midazolam	Hyoscine Hydrobromide	Hyoscine Butylbromide
Diamorphine		C YES	C YES	C YES	YES	YES	YES	YES
Metoclopramide	C YES		n	NO	n	YES	YES	n
Haloperidol	YES C	n		YES	n	YES	YES	YES
Cyclizine	C YES	NO	YES		YES	C YES	YES	YES
Levomepromazine	YES	n	n	YES		YES	YES	YES
Midazolam	YES	YES	YES	C YES	YES		YES	YES
Hyoscine Hydrobromide	YES	YES	YES	YES	YES	YES		n
Hyoscine Butylbromide	YES	n	YES	YES	YES	YES	n	

C = caution at higher concentrations

n = generally not a clinically useful combination (same group of drug or counteracting effects)

scription of drugs to achieve improvement in symptom management. If drug dosages need to be altered, the syringe should be recharged with the new prescription. Do not use a change in rate of delivery, since alteration of the rate will:

- deliver *all* of the drugs at an increased or decreased rate;
- alter the time of next recharge of the syringe and may lead to times without infusion if district nurses are planning visits at the same time each day;
- potentially lead to an overdosage (or underdosage) if the rate is not checked and reset at each syringe recharge;
- make it more difficult to calculate the actual dose of each drug the patient is receiving daily.

Problem preventing and solving

Care of the infusion

Nurses should check regularly:

- for signs of irritation or inflammation at the injection site;
- for evidence of leakage at the various connections;
- that the driver is working (light flashing/intermittent motor noise);
- that the set rate is correct;
- for signs of crystallization or precipitation (cloudy);
- that the tubing is not kinked.

Infusion-site irritation

Should there be persistent problems with irritation at the injection site, consider:

- reducing the concentration of drugs (i.e. larger volume);
- changing the drug; or consider an alternative route (some drugs are much more irritant than others);
- mixing drugs with 0.9% saline (if miscible) to make the infusion isotonic;
- using a Teflon cannula;
- adding hydrocortisone 50 mg or dexamethasone 1 mg to the infusion;
- priming the infusion site with 1500 units of hyaluronidase. This is an enzyme that breaks down connective tissue locally and increases diffusion.

Case history exercise: some thoughts on the plan of management for Jane

In addition to your communication, history, and empathy skills you will need to have the following knowledge and skills to manage Jane effectively:

- medical management of bowel obstruction (see p. 80);

- safe use of the Graseby syringe driver for SC infusion;

- calculation of the correct dose of diamorphine. For Jane, replacement of her sustained release morphine requires 30 mg of diamorphine (40 mg × 2/3). Because she is in pain, she will require a stat SC dose (1/6th total daily dose = 5 mg) and possibly a 30% increase in the total opioid dose (i.e. consider increasing to 40 mg/24 h);

- use of anti-emetics by SC infusion (e.g. cyclizine 150 mg/24 h);

- effective prescribing of the multiple drugs that may be required to manage her symptoms;

- effective identification of other needs (physical, psychological, social, financial, spiritual, practical, etc.);

- how to access specialist advice and support and interventions for you and for Jane and her family;

- how to facilitate discussion with Jane and her husband about the future and to answer their questions and address their concerns;

- optimal discharge planning, including:
  - district nurses to access a Graseby syringe driver in the community and change the infusion daily;
  - access to unusual drugs such as octreotide;
  - liaison with Jane's GP about the current situation and appropriate planning for future potential problems (e.g. referral to community palliative care team/hospice to avoid unwanted hospital admissions).

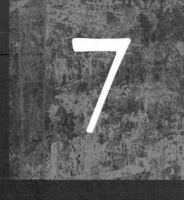

7

CHAPTER 7

Regulations and statutory duties: some rules

◆ Introduction *103*

◆ Prescribing controlled drugs *103*

◆ 'Unlicensed' drug use *106*

◆ Getting money for patients *106*

◆ Death verification *107*

◆ Death certification *107*

◆ Cremation form *109*

CHAPTER 7

Regulations and statutory duties: some rules

Introduction

If you are reading this book cover to cover you should, by now, have a pretty good idea of how to 'do palliative care' well. However, there a few rules you need to know, including:

● prescribing controlled drugs (e.g. strong opioids) and unlicensed drugs;

● how you can help patients get money;

● administrative duties after death.

Familiarity with these is important. Errors made here can have a significant impact on patients or families. Others are more an inconvenience to you and others, but all are a cause for embarrassment.

Prescribing controlled drugs

All strong opioids come under the Misuse of Drugs Regulations 1985. To you, the prescriber, this means that whenever you provide a patient with prescrip-

CONTROLLED DRUGS
Buprenorphine
Codeine injection
Dihydrocodeine injection
Dextromoramide
Diamorphine
Dipipanone
Morphine (> 10 mg in 5 ml strength)
Morphine solid and injectable forms
Fentanyl
Hydromorphone
Methadone
Pentazocine
Pethidine
Phenazocine

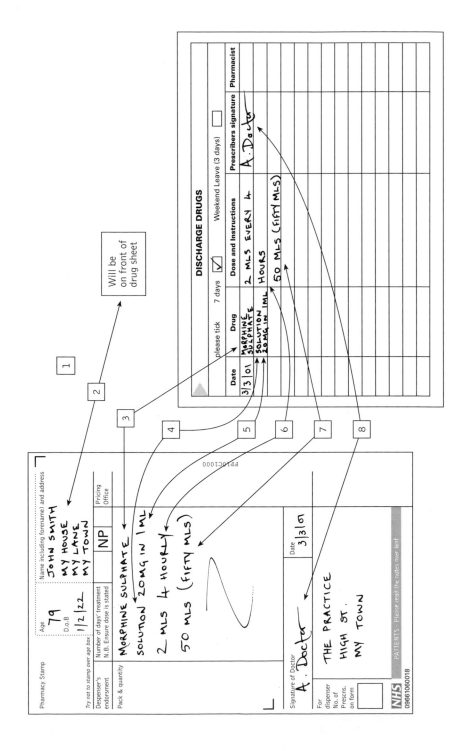

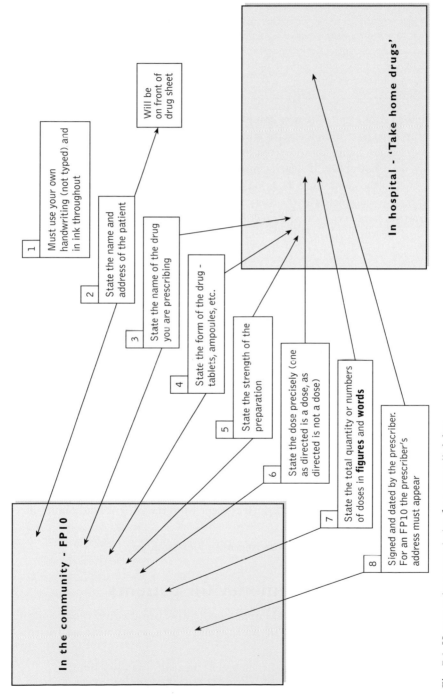

Fig. 7.1 How to write a prescription for a controlled drug

In hospital - 'Take home drugs'

In the community - FP10

1 Must use your own handwriting (not typed) and in ink throughout

2 State the name and address of the patient

Will be on front of drug sheet

3 State the name of the drug you are prescribing

4 State the form of the drug - tablets, ampoules, etc.

5 State the strength of the preparation

6 State the dose precisely (one as directed is a dose, as directed is not a dose)

7 State the total quantity or numbers of doses in **figures** and **words**

8 Signed and dated by the prescriber. For an FP10 the prescriber's address must appear

---

LEARNING TASK

Ask to borrow a drug chart or prescription pad and practise filling it in by writing a prescription for diamorphine 30 mg and cyclizine 30 mg over 24 hours. Check you've done it right by showing someone who knows (e.g. pharmacist or doctor).

---

tion for a strong opioid to take home (on discharge from hospital or in the community) you have to follow certain rules. These are outlined in Fig. 7.1. While the drugs are being administered by ward staff in hospital, then these same rules need not apply. If district nurses are administering strong opioids to patients in the community (e.g. via a syringe driver), then the prescriber will also have to complete the necessary nursing documentation. This makes sure the nurses have very clear and precise advice on how to administer the drug, a process for which you will hold some responsibility.

'Unlicensed' drug use

Prescribing practice in palliative care is an evolving process. By applying existing knowledge, considering pharmaceutical properties of drugs and good, old-fashioned common sense; a palliative care formulary has developed that means that many drugs are used in a way that they were not licensed for. This need not be a problem; doctors are allowed to prescribe in this way. But we have to act reasonably and take responsibility for our actions. Prescribing a drug 'off licence' is fine if it is established practice or if, on balance, the risk to the patient would be generally viewed as low. However, if we use a drug in this way and the cost/benefit ratio to the patient is debatable, then we need to be more cautious. In such circumstances it is wise to:

- record in the patient's notes the reasons for the decision to prescribe 'off licence';
- whenever possible, gain informed consent from the patient (and family if appropriate);
- inform other professionals to avoid misunderstandings.

Getting money for patients

For many, sickness has financial implications; either because they can no longer work and/or they have to buy in care at home. There are various ways patients can receive financial aid:

- the State (e.g. sickness benefit, incapacity benefit, disability living allowance, attendance allowance, invalid care allowance, etc);

- private insurance schemes;
- charitable giving (Macmillan Cancer Relief, local charities).

Each of these may require documentary evidence from you as a doctor. Often, much of the application process is handled by others (e.g. patient, family, social worker, nurse), and it often requires little from a doctor. Usually you have to complete a form, which is self-explanatory. Remember that you need signed consent from the patient before you can pass confidential information to a third party. Even if you are filling a form so the patient gets the money they are asking for!

However, many potential claimants miss out because no one thought about their eligibility and they were unaware of what they were entitled to. Knowing the range of aid available, allows you to prompt thoughts about financial support in the rest of the team. Asking a social worker or nurse if your patient is eligible for any help, can start a process that makes a very real difference to patients.

More specifically, there are two state benefits that require specific documentation in order for terminally ill patients to claim. Disability living allowance and attendance allowance are usually paid once a patient has been unable to work because of sickness for 6 months. Obviously in palliative care, we are often faced with patients who have a shorter prognosis than this. In such circumstances, you as the doctor can sign a DS1500 form that allows this rule to be wavered and for patients to receive this benefit immediately.

Death verification

Once a patient has died, the death will need to be confirmed. It might be hard to believe, but errors very occasionally happen when verifying death. The consequences of this do not need emphasizing! Also, delays in completing any of the formal after-death procedures can cause considerable distress and inconvenience to relatives. We need to get this right! Figure 7.2 illustrates the procedures around death verification.

Death certification

Once the death has occurred then a death certificate needs to be issued. Only then can the funeral directors and family proceed with their funeral arrangements. The certificate also has a statuary function in that it is legal evidence of cause of death and provides epidemiological data. In order to avoid unnecessary delay for the bereaved, it is helpful if you complete the death certificate as soon as is practicable.

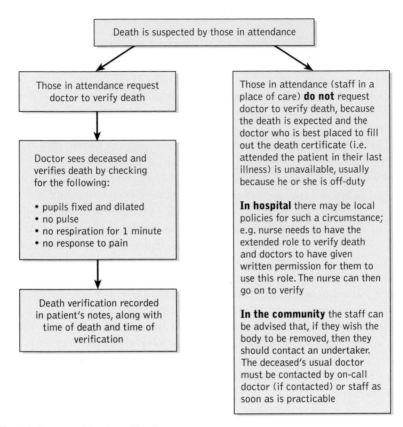

Fig. 7.2 Process of death verification

The doctor who attended the deceased during their last illness is best placed to complete the death certificate, but he or she can only issue a death certificate if he/she is sure:

● that they the cause of death is known;
● that the patient had been seen by a doctor in the last 14 days;
● that there are:
  – no suspicious circumstances
  – no evidence of violence
  – no links with an accident
  – no evidence of self-neglect or neglect by others (including medical care)
  – no links with an abortion
  – no suspicions of suicide
  – no suspicions of the death being linked to an industrial injury/disease
  – no suspicions that the death was related to medical treatment

- no history of fractures
- no evidence of a recent fall;
- that the patient was not detained under the Mental Health Act;
- that the patient was not recently held under police or prison custody;
- that the patient was not in receipt of a war pension or industrial disability pension;
- that the patient had not been operated on recently, or at least that full recovery from anaesthetic was achieved;
- that the admission was not less than 24 hours.

LEARNING EXERCISE

Ask a doctor or the hospital bereavement officer if you could practise writing a death certificate. They may be able to provide you with a set of notes and a certificate, which you can try to complete, getting them to check it afterwards.

If you have any doubt about whether to certify a death or not, then you can check the regulations, which can be found in the front of the death certificate book, or speak to the coroner or his/her officer. The coroner's team are usually very helpful and may allow you to issue a certificate if the query is minor. They can be contacted via the local police station.

The rules around how to fill the death certificate are illustrated in Fig.7.3.

Cremation form

If the deceased is going to be cremated, then it is necessary for two doctors to examine the deceased and make an assessment of the cause of death. This is to make sure that there will be no mistakes regarding any future need to examine the body. The form is in two parts. Part 1 is completed by the doctor who filled in the death certificate, and Part 2 by a second doctor.

THINK POINT

Did you know that the doctor's fee for completing the cremation form is paid by the funeral director, who will then bill the relatives?

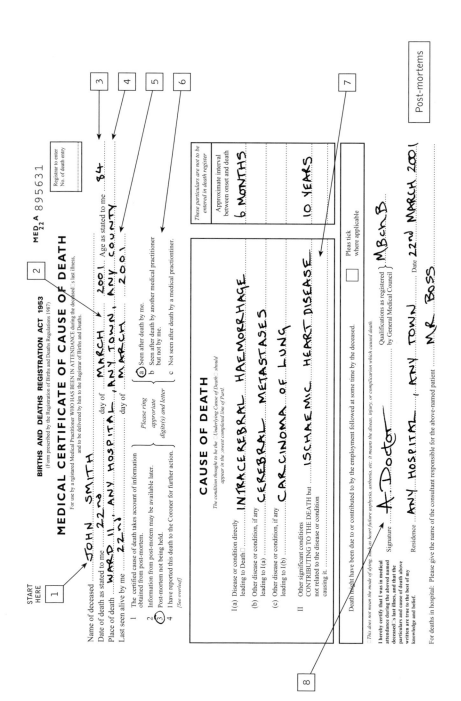

Post-mortems

BIRTHS AND DEATHS REGISTRATION ACT 1953
(Form prescribed by the Registration of Births and Deaths Regulations 1987)

MED A 895631
22

2

MEDICAL CERTIFICATE OF CAUSE OF DEATH

For use by a registered Medical Practitioner WHO HAS BEEN IN ATTENDANCE during the deceased's last illness, and to be delivered by him to the Registrar of Births and Deaths.

Registrar to enter
No. of death entry

START HERE 1

Name of deceased .... JOHN SMITH

Date of death as stated to me ... 22nd ..... day of ... MARCH ... 2001. Age as stated to me ... 84

Place of death ... WARD 11, ANY HOSPITAL, ANY TOWN, ANY COUNTY .. 3

Last seen alive by me .... 22nd .... day of ... MARCH ... 2001. 4

1   The certified cause of death takes account of information obtained from post-mortem.
2   Information from post-mortem may be available later.
③ Post-mortem not being held.
4   I have reported this death to the Coroner for further action.
[See overleaf]

{ *Please ring appropriate digit(s) and letter*

ⓐ Seen after death by me.
b Seen after death by another medical practitioner but not by me. 5
c Not seen after death by a medical practitioner. 6

CAUSE OF DEATH

The condition thought to be the *Underlying Cause of Death   should appear in the lowest completed line of Part1.*

I (a) Disease or condition directly leading to Death☐... INTRACEREBRAL HAEMORRHAGE

(b) Other disease or condition, if any leading to I(a) ... CEREBRAL METASTASES

(c) Other disease or condition, if any leading to I(b) ... CARCINOMA OF LUNG

II   Other significant conditions CONTRIBUTING TO THE DEATH but not related to the disease or condition causing it. ... ISCHAEMIC HEART DISEASE 7

These particulars are not to be entered in death register

Approximate interval between onset and death

6 MONTHS

10 YEARS

☐ Pleas tick where applicable

Death might have been due to or contributed to by the employment followed at some time by the deceased.

☐ Pleas tick where applicable

☐This does not mean the mode of dying, such as heart failure asphyxia, asthenia, etc: it means the diseas, injury, or complication which caused death.

I hereby certify that I was in medical attendance during the above named deceased's last illness, and that the particulars and cause of death above written are true to the best of my knowledge and belief.

Signature ... A. Doctor 8

Qualifications as registered } M.B.ch.B
by General Medical Council }

Residence ... ANY HOSPITAL, ANY TOWN ...... Date 22nd MARCH 2001

For deaths in hospital: Please give the name of the consultant responsible for the above-named patient ...... MR BOSS

START HERE

1 Full name of patient

2 Date of death

3 Age of patient

4 Place of death (ward and hospital)

5 Last seen alive by me

DEATH CERTIFICATE (COPY)

6 Circle 1, 2, 3, or 4 and a, b, or c; depending on the circumstances

Post-mortem

If the coroner is performing a post-mortem, you will not be completing the certificate. However, if the relatives consent and a post-mortem is thought to be valuable ('hospital post-mortem'), then you will need to ring 1 or 2.

9 Complete;
- Counterfoil; unlike the rest of the certificate, you can use abbreviations here
- 'Notice to informants.' This is pinned to the envelope containing the completed certificate and handed to the relatives.

8 Complete the form by:
- Signing it
- Print your name beneath your signature
- Residence can be stated as the hospital
- Print the name of the consultant

Cause of death

7 You must try and complete this to the best of your knowledge and belief. Work your way through the patient's history until you reach the underlying cause of death. Unlike the example given here, you don't have to write something in 1b or 1c if clinically there is nothing to write. Do not put mode of death as a cause (e.g. coma, cardiac arrest, etc.)

1 (a) Intracerebral haemorrhage
1 (b) Cerebral metastases
1 (c) Carcinoma of lung

Time

Often very hard to work out. Just complete as closely as possible (e.g. 6 months, 10 years)

7.3 Completed death certificate

SUMMARY BOX

There are administrative duties required of doctors and we need to be efficient at them. These include:

◆ prescribing strong opioids;

◆ prescribing drugs 'off licence';

◆ getting money for patients;

◆ verifying and certifying death;

◆ completing the cremation form.

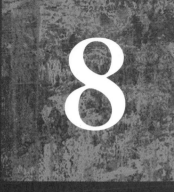

8

CHAPTER 8

Further information about palliative care and useful resources

◆ Specialist palliative care services *115*

◆ Addresses and websites *119*

CHAPTER 8

Further information about palliative care and useful resources

Specialist palliative care services

Palliative care in the UK, either in hospital or the community, is supported by an array of specialist services. The roles of specialist palliative care services are:

- to be a resource of specialist expertise, services, and equipment;
- to provide education;
- to train specialist practitioners;
- to undertake research.

If you are in any doubt about any aspect of palliative care, use them. They are there to help you provide the best care for your patients. Get to know those that are local to you, how to make contact with them, and refer patients to them.

The components of a specialist palliative care service

Because of the historically unplanned provision of palliative care services (often provided by charitable organizations), the precise model of specialist palliative care services will differ between districts. In general, the elements available for you to find for your patients should be as follows.

The hospice

A hospice provides a service for people with advanced, progressive, life-threatening diseases. Hospices may be NHS or charitable. They may provide all or any of inpatient and outpatient care, day care, and care in the patient's home. This will vary from hospice to hospice; for instance, not all hospices will have inpatient beds. Most will also provide bereavement care of some form.

Home care

For many patients, a specialist nurse (sometime called a Macmillan Nurse, see below) working in the community alongside the primary healthcare team is the only component of specialist palliative care they will need. If the specialist home-care nurse works from a hospice or specialist palliative care unit he or she will provide the contact point for the other components of the specialist service (e.g. medical advice, access to inpatient services).

Some home-care teams will work 9 a.m. to 5 p.m. Monday through Friday, other teams will provide a 24-hour service 7 days a week.

Hospice at home

These teams are a relatively new development and are not available in all health districts. Their aim is to provide 24-hour care in the patient's own home in order to avoid unwanted admission in the last days of a patient's life. They may sometimes be called Respite at Home Teams or Rapid Response Teams. Increasingly, patients needing intensive nursing care are being managed in their own homes.

Inpatient care

Inpatient care may be provided in designated palliative care beds, staffed by a specialist multiprofessional team, in several different settings:

- in specialist palliative care units or hospices;
- in palliative care beds in acute hospitals, community hospitals, or nursing homes.

It is the team of professionals, their knowledge, skills, and philosophy of care, not the actual place of care, that comprises specialist inpatient care (i.e. a hospice is not solely a building).

Patients may need admission for:

- terminal care when continued care at home is not possible and hospital or nursing home care is inappropriate because of the patient's and/or carer's specific needs;
- short stays for complex symptom control;
- respite care in order to allow continued care in the community through adequate support of the carer;
- rehabilitation for patients with late-stage disease who require particular skills from staff, working together rapidly for realistic, achievable objectives outlined by the patient and the carer.

Day care

The day-care unit can provide support for patients and respite to carers. It normally offers:

- an environment of security, understanding, and mutual support, aiming to normalize and have control and choices in living with an advancing illness;
- promotion of rehabilitation and help towards independence in activities of daily living;

- support and therapy in the form of social activities, the relief of isolation and depression, and the general enhancement of well being through, for example, chiropody, hair care, aromatherapy, and massage;
- some nursing measures, including dressings and help with stoma care;
- assessment, monitoring, advice, and intervention in symptom control;
- access to medical advice;
- discussion of diagnosis and prognosis.

Outpatient clinics

- Clinics may be held in hospital specialist units/hospices or community health clinics.
- Referral is made doctor to doctor.
- Most provide general assessment, advice, intervention, and monitoring of physical and non-physical symptoms.
- Specific clinics may be provided by doctors and other healthcare professionals for the management of lymphoedema and dyspnoea and access to complementary therapies, psychological support in early disease, nerve blocks, and other interventional pain management techniques.

Hospital support teams

The hospital support team works mainly in an advisory capacity alongside other hospital professionals, e.g. in oncology, surgery, general medicine. The team requires a multiprofessional membership, similar to teams working in the community. Their role is:

- assessment of patient needs, e.g. symptom control, counselling, quality of life;
- specialist advice on symptom control and other needs;
- support, information, and advice to patients, families, informal carers;
- support, information, and advice to professional carers in hospital;
- education of professionals;
- promotion of continuity of care upon discharge of patient;
- research.

Bereavement support

The role of this service is to assess the need for support for carers and to offer this support in a carefully monitored and supervised way. Ideally, this work should begin before the death of the patient to prevent problems, particularly with those at risk of an abnormal or difficult bereavement.

The service offered may comprise telephone contact, bereavement visiting, attendance at a bereavement group, bereavement counselling to individuals and families, and referral on to other agencies. Some units may offer specific services for bereaved children.

Palliative care nursing services: who does what?

District nurse

District nurses play an important part in domiciliary palliative care. They provide hands-on nursing care, sometimes visiting the patients up to three times a day. The availability of night district nurses services varies from area to area. They are contacted either via the GP surgery or their central base.

Role:

- assessment of need;
- general nursing care (e.g. dressings, pressure area care, bowel care, etc.);
- emotional support to patients and their families;
- health education and advice to patients and families;
- is often the key worker for patients and families in the community;
- organizing equipment (e.g. mattresses, commodes, syringe drivers, etc.);
- co-ordinating and accessing other services (GP, Marie Curie nurses, hospital nurses).

Marie Curie nurse

These nurses (of various grades) are organized and funded in part by the nationwide Marie Curie charity. They provide hands-on nursing care, staying with the patient for a number of hours, often overnight. This important service allows many patients to be managed at home, so avoiding inappropriate admissions for nursing care. They are contacted through a designated agency.

Role:

- 'hands-on' general nursing care;
- emotional support to patients and their families.

Specialist palliative care nurse

Also known as Macmillan nurse, hospice home care nurse, or continuing care nurse. These nurses have added to their basic and post-registration education, a period of specific palliative care training. Some will be termed as 'Macmillan nurses' in recognition of the charitable organization who funded their initial 3 years. They usually work as part of a multiprofessional specialist team. They are contacted by referral to the hospital team, hospice, or specialist community service.

Role:

- will assess the palliative care needs of patients;
- bring specialist knowledge (e.g. symptom control, nursing care, ethical issues, etc.);
- provide emotional support to patient, carers, and staff;
- may access hospice-based services (e.g. day care, additional aids, volunteers, etc.);
- some will provide bereavement follow-up;
- provide education.

Addresses and websites

Information about palliative care services

International Association for Hospice and Palliative Care
Liliana De Lima MHA, c/o UT MD Anderson Cancer Center, 1515 Holcombe Blvd. Box 08, Houston, Texas 77030, USA
http://www.hospicecare.com

Macmillan Cancer Relief
89 Albert Embankment, London SE1 7UQ, UK
Tel.: 020 7840 7840
http://www.macmillan.org.uk

Marie Curie Cancer Care
89 Albert Embankment, London SE1 7TP, UK
Tel.: 020 7599 7729
http://www.mariecurie.org.uk/

National Council for Hospices and Specialist Palliative Care Services
First Floor, 34–44 Britannia Street, London WC1X 9JG, UK
Tel.: 020 7520 8299
http://www.hospice-spc-council.org.uk/indexf.htm

Scottish Partnership Agency for Palliative and Cancer Care
1A Cambridge Street, Edinburgh EH1 2DY, UK
Tel.: 0131 229 0538
http://www.spapcc.demon.co.uk/

The Association for Palliative Medicine of Great Britain and Ireland
11, Westwood Road, Southampton SO17 1DL, UK
Tel.: 01703 672888
http://www.palliative-medicine.org/

The Hospice Information Service
51–59 Lawrie Park Road, London SE26 6DZ, UK
Tel.: 020 8778 9252
http://www.hospiceinformation.co.uk

Information about cancer

BACUP – British Association of Cancer United Patients
http://www.cancerbacup.org.uk

CancerHelp UK – University of Birmingham
http://medweb.bham.ac.uk/cancerhelp/indexy.html

National Cancer Institute (USA)
http://www.cancernet.nci.nih.gov

The Information line (Cancer Relief Macmillan)
Tel.: 0845 601 6161

University of Newcastle, guide to internet resources for cancer
http://www.cancerindex.org/clinks1.htm

Information about non-malignant advanced, progressive, life-threatening diseases

Alzheimer's Disease Society
Gordon House, 10 Greencoat Place, London SW1P 1PH, UK
Tel.: 020 7306 0606
http://www.alzheimers.org.uk/

Motor Neurone Disease Association of Australia
http://home.vicnet.net.au/~mndaust/

Motor Neurone Disease Association of England, Wales and Northern Ireland
PO Box 246, Northampton NN1 2PR, UK
Tel.: 01604 250505
Helpline: 08457 626262
http://www.mndassociation.org/indx.html

Multiple Sclerosis Society
The MS National Centre, 372 Edgware Road, London NW2 6ND, UK
Tel.: 020 84380700
http://www.mssociety.org.uk/

Parkinson's Disease Society of the United Kingdom
215 Vauxhall Bridge Road, London SW1V 1EJ, UK
Tel.: 020 7931 8080
Helpline (available Monday to Friday, 10.00 a.m. to 4.00 p.m.):
020 7388 5798
http://www.shef.ac.uk/misc/groups/epda/parkuk.htm

Scottish Motor Neurone Disease Association
76 Firhill Road, Glasgow G20 7BA, UK
0141 9451077
http://www.scotmnd.org.uk

Terrence Higgins Trust
52–54 Gray's Inn Road, London WC 1X 8JU, UK
Tel.: 020 7831 0330
http://www.tht.org.uk/

Information about palliative care and pain

BMJ-collected resources on palliative medicine since 1994
http://www.bmj.com/cgi/collection/palliative_medicine

European Journal of Palliative Care
http://www.ejpc.co.uk

Helpful links to palliative care (University of Dundee)
http://www.dundee.ac.uk/meded/help/sectionb

International Association for the Study of Pain (IASP)
http://www.halycon.com/iasp

Palliative care issues
http://www.e-bpm

Palliativedrugs.com—online palliative care resource
http://www.palliativedrugs.com/

Palliative Medicine, journal
http://www.arnoldpublishers.com/Journals/Journpages/02692163.htm

Progress in Palliative Care, journal
http://www.leeds.ac.uk/lmi/ppc/ppcmain.html

**Shaare Zedek Cancer Pain and Palliative Care Reference Database:
Roxanne laboratories**
http://www.roxane.com/

Information about death and dying

Death and Dying
http://dying.about.com/health/dying/mbody.htm

Natural Death Centre; woodland burials, cardboard coffins, green funerals
http://www.naturaldeath.org.uk/

References

Chapter 1

1. World Health Organization (1990). *Cancer pain relief and palliative care*, Technical Report Series: 804. World Health Organization, Geneva.
2. Saunders, C. (1967). The care of the terminal stages of cancer. *Annals of the Royal College of Surgeons of England*, 41 (Suppl.), 162–169.
3. Kubler-Ross, E. (1969). *On death and dying*. Macmillan, New York.
4. Parkes, C. M. (1991). *Bereavement: studies of grief in adult life*, (2nd edn). Penguin, London.
5. Hinton, J. (1972). *Dying* (2nd edn). Penguin, London.
6. Robinson, I. and Hunter, M. (1998). *Motor neurone disease*. Routledge, London.

Chapter 2

1. Faulkner, A. and Maguire, P. (1994). *Talking to cancer patients and their relatives*. Oxford University Press, Oxford.

Chapter 3

1. Kubler-Ross, E. (1969). *On death and dying*. Macmillan, New York.
2. Saunders, C. M. (1967). *The management of terminal illness*. Hospital Medicine Publications, London.
3. Glaser, B. G. and Strauss, A. L. (1965). *Awareness of dying*. Adeline, Chicago.
4. Timmermans, S. (1994). Dying awareness: the theory of awareness revisted. *Social Health and illness*, 16, 322–37.
5. Balint, M. (1963). *The doctor, his patient and the illness*, (2nd edn). Churchill, London.

Chapter 4

1. Kramer, H. and Kramer, K. (1993). *Conversations at midnight*. William Morrow, New York.
2. Porter, R. (1990). In *The ruffian on the stairs*, ed. R. Dinnage, p. 210. Penguin, London.
3. Gillon, R. (1994). Medical ethics: Four principles plus attention to scope. *British Medical Journal*, 309, 184–8.

4. British Medical Association (1995). *Advance statements about medical treatment: code of practice with explanatory notes.* Report of the British Medical Association. BMJ Publishing Group, London.

5. Website of Resuscitation Council (UK) www.resus.org.uk.

Chapter 5

1. Ahmedzai, S. (1982). Dying in hospital: the resident's viewpoint. *British Medical Journal*, **285**, 712–14.

2. Mills, M., Davies, H. T. O. and Macrae, W. A. (1994). Care of dying patients in hospital. *British Medical Journal*, **309**, 583–6.

3. World Health Organization (1996). *Cancer pain relief.* WHO, Geneva.

Further reading

Chapter 4

Ethics and ethical dilemmas

Randall, F. and Downie, R. S. (1999). *Palliative Care Ethics: A Companion for Specialists*, (2nd edn). Oxford University Press, Oxford.

Roy, D. J. and MacDonald, N. (1998). Ethical issues in palliative care. In Doyle, D., Hanks, G. W. C. and MacDonald N. eds. Oxford Textbook of Palliative Medicine.

Cardiopulmonary resuscitation

British Medical Association (2001). *Decisions relating to cardiopulmonary resuscitation*. A statement from the BMA and RCN in association with the resuscitation council (UK).

Joint Working party between National Council for Hospice and Specialist Palliative Care Services and Ethics Committee of the Association for Palliative Medicine of Great Britain and Ireland (1997). *Ethical decision-making in palliative care: cardiopulmonary resuscitation (CPR) for people who are terminally ill*. National Council for Hospice and Specialist palliative care Services, London.

Stewart, K. (1997). Discussing cardiopulmonary resuscitation with patients and relatives. In *Communication skills in Medicine*, (ed. Hind, C. R. K.). BMJ Publishing Group, London.

Withdrawing and withholding life-sustaining treatments

British Medical Association (1999). *Withholding and withdrawing life sustaining treatments*. Report of the British Medical Association. BMJ Publishing Group, London.

Joint Working party between National Council for Hospice and Specialist Palliative Care Services and Ethics Committee of the Association for Palliative Medicine of Great Britain and Ireland (1997). *Ethical decision-making in palliative care: artificial hydration for people who are terminally ill*. National Council for Hospice and Specialist palliative care Services, London.

Chapter 5

Bauby, Jean-Dominique (1997). *The diving-bell and the butterfly*. HarperCollins Publishers Ltd.

British National Formulary

Doyle, D., Hanks, G., and MacDonald, N. (1997). *Oxford textbook of palliative medicine*, (2nd edn). Oxford University Press, Oxford.

Faull, C., Carter, Y., and Woof, R. (1998). *Handbook of palliative care*, Blackwell Science, Oxford.

Regnard, C., and Tempest, S. (1998). *A guide to symptom relief in advanced disease*, (4th edn). Hochland and Hochland, Hale.

Twycross, R., Wilcock, A., and Thorp, S. (1998). *Palliative care formulary*. Radcliffe Medical Press, Abingdon.

Spence, C., and Johnston, P. G. (2001) *Oncology – An Oxford Core Text*. Oxford University Press, Oxford.

Chapter 6

David, J. (1992). A survey of the use of syringe drivers in Marie Curie Centres. *European Journal of Cancer Care* 1, 23–8.

Dover, S. B. (1987). Syringe driver in terminal care. *British Medical Journal*, 294, 553–5.

Johnson, J. (1998). The syringe driver. In *Handbook of palliative care*, (ed. Faull, C., Carter, Y., and Woof, R.), pp. 356–75. Blackwell Science, Oxford.

Nicholson, H. (1986). The success of the syringe driver. *Nursing Times* 9 July, 49–51.

O'Neill, W. M. (1994). Subcutaneous infusions—a medical last rite. *Palliative Medicine* 8, 91–3.

How much palliative medicine do you need to learn?

One of the hardest things about learning is deciding what you need to know—how do you know what you don't know? For the student with their eyes on the next exam, the answer to this question is usually—whatever the teacher decides or, more honestly, what questions am I likely to be asked? For the practising clinician, learning is less driven by exams and more by our professional ethic of wanting to do our best and continue to develop our knowledge, skills, and attitude; although increasingly, revalidation is going to, require us to demonstrate competence. To help you appreciate the range of topic areas expected of you, the Association for Palliative Medicine has devised a curriculum for undergraduates. We have given this here so that you can assess your areas of strength and weakness. As a core list of things to know, it is also useful for doctors in training.

How to use this questionnaire

Go through the curriculum and rate your ability in a particular area by ticking the most appropriate box according to how you think you might do in an exam. Once completed you can then identify areas of weakness and consider how to fill this gap. You may find that there are large areas where you feel underconfident, don't worry about this. This book will have many of the answers for you and you will pick up many other things in your training. You might need to look up things elsewhere, we've usually tried to give you guidance on this through the text of the book.

To help you further we have devised a scoring system which helps you identify broader areas of strengths; be that needing to know more, being more able to do certain things, or having a greater awareness of certain issues.

Example

Topic area	Imagine being asked a question about this in an exam, how would you do?					Comments
	Perform Awfully ← → Perform Brilliantly					
	1	2	3	4	5	
Disease process						*I knew this was true, but I'm not clear which cancers are curable. I'll check this out when I do my oncology module in the 4th year.*
1 Be aware that cancer may be curable and does not mean a terminal illness			✓			

The questionnaire

Topic area	Imagine being asked a question about this in an exam, how would you do?					Comments
	Perform Awfully ← → Perform Brilliantly					
	1	2	3	4	5	
Disease process						
1 Be aware that cancer may be curable and does not always mean a terminal illness						
2 Understand that the principles of palliative medicine are also applicable to people with a wide variety of life-threatening illnesses						
3 Understand the concept of re-evaluation as the disease progresses (i.e. knowing the best way to follow people up)						
Symptom control						
4 Understand that symptoms can be caused by the disease, treatment, co-morbidity, or disease complication						
5 Know how to take a pain history well						
6 Diagnosis of different types of pain—pain can be categorized, do you know any commonly used classifications?						
7 Appreciate that pain is not just a physical phenomenon, it is also social, psychological, spiritual?						

Topic area		Imagine being asked a question about this in an exam, how would you do?					Comments
		Perform Awfully ← → Perform Brilliantly					
		1	2	3	4	5	
8 The concept of opioid-sensitive pain. An understanding of the array of drugs used for pain							
9 How to monitor the response to treatment							
10 Sore mouth	For each of these symptoms think of all the causes you can, how you would diagnose them, and the management options you know of						
11 Candidiasis							
12 Anorexia							
13 Nausea and vomiting							
14 Constipation							
15 Diarrhoea							
16 Dyspnoea							
17 Cough							
18 Hiccup							
19 Anxiety and fear							
20 Depression							
21 Acute confusional state							

Topic area	Imagine being asked a question about this in an exam, how would you do? Perform Awfully ←→ Perform Brilliantly					Comments
	1	2	3	4	5	
Pharmacology						
22 Analgesics can be classified into different groups—do you know how?						
23 Which drugs are commonly used for the control of symptoms, usual frequency of administration, typical doses, and common adverse effects						
24 Various routes of administration of different drugs and when each is appropriate						
25 The indications for a syringe driver						
Psychosocial aspects						
26 Be able to assess differing perceptions and expectations of disease and treatment among the various family members						
27 Be able to draw up a family tree						
Communication skills						
28 How to listen to patients effectively						
29 How to assess the patient's knowledge of the diagnosis and prognosis						
30 How to break bad news						
31 How to give information at appropriate times						
32 Dealing with difficult questions (e.g. 'how long have I got?')						
33 Eliciting and responding to the fears of patients and their family in a way that helps them						
34 Enabling the patients to make their own choices for themselves						

Topic area	Imagine being asked a question about this in an exam, how would you do?					Comments
	Perform Awfully ←→ Perform Brilliantly					
	1	2	3	4	5	
Psychosocial responses						
35 Understand responses to loss and that these may manifest themselves normally at various times and are a form of grief						
36 Understand the importance of hope, and that this may mean setting goals other than cure						
Sexuality						
37 Understand the patient's perception of their sexuality, including body image and the effect of disease on this						
38 The need to allow the patient and family to express affection						
Grief						
39 Know the common patterns of bereavement						
40 Be able to support a bereaved person						
Awareness of personal feelings						
41 Be aware and respond to emotional stress in oneself and others in the team; and the potential dangers of this stress in patient care						
42 Recognize how you would seek help when stressed yourself						
43 Cope with feelings of guilt in yourself and others as a response to your patient's plight						
44 Recognize how our own belief systems influence how we behave and the dangers in projecting them on others						

Topic area	Imagine being asked a question about this in an exam, how would you do? Perform Awfully ←→ Perform Brilliantly					Comments
	1	2	3	4	5	
Religious and cultural aspects						
45 Know when you need to ask for help when responding to spiritual needs of patients						
46 Be able to recognize the importance of religious and cultural influences, including language, on all aspects of palliative care						
Ethical aspects						
47 How to appreciate the goals and priorities important to patients						
48 How to negotiate and agree management plans with patients						
49 How to always tell the truth to a patient when asked, even if this goes against the wishes of a third party (e.g. family member)						
50 Letting patients know everything *they* need to and not to withhold information inappropriately						
51 Respecting a patient's wish to decline treatment						
52 How treatment should never be prescribed with the primary aim of killing a patient						
53 That we should not treat patients if it means prolonging their natural death						
54 How to handle a request for euthanasia						
55 Recognize the dangers in making judgements about patients according to your view of their age and pre-morbidity						

Topic area	Imagine being asked a question about this in an exam, how would you do?					Comments
	Perform Awfully ← → Perform Brilliantly					
	1	2	3	4	5	
56 How to weigh up the pros and cons of a situation with patients						
57 Understand that the patient has the right to the highest standard of care within the resources available. And appreciate how these decisions are made and communicated						
Teamwork						
58 Value the skills and contributions of others, both medical and non-medical, to palliative care situations. You need to know which professionals (especially specialist palliative care in the hospital and community) can help, and to take appropriate advice from them						
59 Understand how teams work best together and your role in this						
Organizational aspects						
60 How to certify death						
61 When and how to liaise with the coroner's officer						
62 Cremation regulations						
63 Procedures for relatives following a death and how cultural influences affect this						
64 Grants, funds, and allowances for the terminally ill						

Overall scoring

Knowledge (K)		Skills (S)		Attitude (A)	
Question	Your score (out of 5)	Question	Your score (out of 5)	Question	Your score (out of 5)
1		5		7	
2		26		34	
3		27		37	
4		28		38	
6		29		41	
8		30		42	
9		31		43	
10		32		44	
11		22		46	
12		40		49	
13		47		50	
14		48		51	
15		59		52	
16		60		53	
17		61		55	
18		62		56	
19		63		57	
20		64		58	
21					
22					
23					
24					
25					
35					
36					
39					
45					
54					

Total (K) (out of 140) ☐   **Total (S)** (out of 90) ☐   **Total (A)** (out of 90) ☐

Scoring examples

Now plot your total scores for knowledge, skills, and attitude along the corresponding axes. Then join the marks by drawing an oval. From here you can make some assessment of broad strengths or weaknesses.

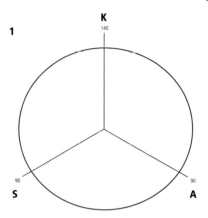

1

Your are either over-confident or are about to apply to be a consultant in palliative medicine!

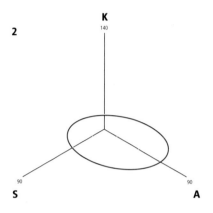

2

You seem strong attitudinally and with some skills, but perhaps you need to focus more getting to know more facts. Read the chapters on symptom control and test yourself with some of the exercises

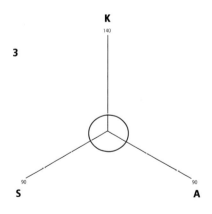

3

You are either grossly underestimating your abilities and need to prove to yourself you are better than this by doing some of the exercises in this book, or you need to speak to your personal tutor!

Drugs you will use frequently for symptom management

A wide range of drugs is available for symptom management. We suggest that you gain familiarity and a good working knowledge of a relatively small group that you may need on a frequent basis. You need to know when to use them, common and important side-effects, cautions and interactions, and methods of administration. You should use other textbooks to familiarize yourself with their pharmacology.

Analgesics

Step 1   Non-opioids

- Paracetamol
- Ibuprofen
- Diclofenac

Step 2   Opioids for mild to moderate pain

- Codeine

Step 3   Opioids for severe pain

- Morphine
- Diamorphine

Adjuvants

- Amitriptyline
- Carbamazepine

Antiemetics

- Metoclopramide
- Cyclizine

Anticholinergics

- Hyoscine butylbromide and hydrobromide

Steroids

- Dexamethasone
- Prednisolone

Sedatives

- Midazolam
- Haloperidol
- Levomepromazine

Laxatives

- Senna

Index

5-HT 67–8
abdominal pain 67
acceptance 35
addiction 7
adjuvant analgesics 77–9
advance statements about treatments 48–9
advanced disease 8, 9, 64
alcoholic cirrhosis 40
allodynia 77
amitriptyline 79
analgesic 35, 74, 89
  adjuvant 77–9
  ladder 72–4, 77
  non-opioid 72, 74
  strong opioid 75
  weak opioid 74–5
anger 24, 31, 32, 34, 35
anorexia 64
anti emetics 67, 68, 75, 89, 96, 99
antibiotics 59, 68
anticholinergic drugs 89, 96
anticipation 65–6
anticonvulsants 79
antidepressants, tricyclic 79
antitussive measures 68
anxiety 35, 64
aspiration pneumonia 68
assessment 66–8
Association for Palliative Medicine of Great
  Britain and Ireland 11
attendance allowance 107
attention to detail 18–19, 70

bad news, breaking of 24
Balint, M. 36
bargaining 34
barriers 21–2
  external 38–9
  internal 39–40
Bauby, J.-P. 69–70
behaviour 32, 33, 34
benzodiazepines 68
bereavement support 117–18
bisacodyl suppositories 80
blocking 21–2
boost button 94–5

British Medical Association 48, 54
buprenorphine 103
burnout 40–1, 50

cancer 8, 53, 64, 68, 71
  breast 66
  lung 3
  ovarian 90
    related pain 7, 73
carbamazepine 79
cardiopulmonary resuscitation 51–5
case histories 11–12, 99
  cancer 66
  motor neurone disease 9, 11–12
  multiple sclerosis 53, 58–9
  Parkinson's disease 47, 58
  renal cell carcinoma 31
catheterization 67
charitable organizations 107
chemotherapy 67
chlorpromazine 89
chronic heart disease 8
circulatory problems 8
co-morbidity 67
codeine 74, 103
colleagues 38
communication 16–18, 37–8
  limited 23–5
confidence 22, 39
confusion 64
constipation 64, 67, 83, 90
contexts of awareness 35–6
continuity 70–1
control, loss of 50
controlled drugs 63, 103–6
coronary heart disease 64
cough 68, 82
cremation form 109–12
Cushing, H. 29
cyclizine 80, 81, 96, 97, 99, 106

danthramer 80
dantron 75

day care 116–17
death
  at home 55–6
  certification 107–9
  verification 107
decisions at end of life 45–59
  advance statements about treatments 48–9
  cardiopulmonary resuscitation 51–5
  case histories 58–9
  death as universal certainty 45–6
  dying in place of choice 55–7
  euthanasia 50–1
  life-sustaining treatments 51
  'right' decisions 46–8
dementia 64
denial 34
depression 35, 40, 50, 64
dexamethasone 79, 80, 96, 98
dextromoramide 103
dextroproxyphene 74
diabetic neuropathy 78
diamorphine 76–7, 95, 96, 97, 103, 106
diarrhoea 83
diazepam 80, 81, 89
diclofenac 89
difficult situations 22–3
dihydrocodeine 74, 103
dipipanone 103
disability living allowance 107
distress 63, 66, 67
district nurse 118
Do-Not-Resuscitate 54–5
domperidone 80, 81, 89
dopamine type 2 receptors 81
drugs 77
  administration see syringe driver
  controlled 103–6
  use, unlicensed 106
DS1500 form 107
dying, stages of 34–5
dysaesthesia 77
dyspnoea 82

emotions 31, 32, 33, 34
  see also anger; anxiety; confusion; denial;
    fear; sadness
empathy 11
enemas 67
epidemiology for the houseman 8–9
ethical considerations 47, 59
ethnic groups 25
Europe 71
euthanasia 24, 50–1
evaluation 66–8

evidence-base 11
evidence-based good practice 47
examination 20–1
explanation 68

family tree 18–19
fatigue 64
Faulkner, A. 21
fear 31, 32, 50
feelings see emotions
fentanyl 103
financial benefits for patients 106–7
fluids see hydration
further information and resources 115–21
  addresses and websites 119–21
  specialist palliative care services 115–19

gabapentin 79
gamma-amino-butyric acid 81
gastric stasis 68
General Medical Council 10
Glaser, B. G. 35
glycerine suppositories 80
goals of palliative care 4–6
good medical practice 10–11

Halford, Sir H. 7
haloperidol 80, 81, 95, 96, 97
heart attacks 8
Hinton, J. 8
Hippocrates 7
histamine type 1 receptors 81
historical background 7
HIV/AIDS 49, 64
Hodgkin's disease 10
home care 115–16
hospice movement 35, 115, 116
hospital support schemes 117
hyaluronidase 98
hydration 51, 53, 59
hydrocortisone 98
hydromorphone 103
hyoscine 81
  butylbromide 80, 96, 97
  hydrobromide 95, 96, 97
hyperaesthesia 77
hyperalgesia 77
hypercalcaemia 67
hyperpathia 77

illness 40
incontinence 64
individualized treatment 68–9
infarction 77
infection 77
information 68
infusion
  care 98
  commencement 93
  lines 59
  preparation 92
  rate 94
  site irritation 98
  and time to take effect 94
inpatient care 116
intramuscular drugs 89
intravenous drugs 89
intravenous lines 59
investigation 20–1

Kramer, H. 45
Kramer, K. 45
Kubler-Ross, E. 8, 34

laxatives 75, 80
legal considerations 47, 49, 59
levomepromazine 81, 95, 96, 97
life-sustaining treatments 51
listening 16–18
local anesthetic 68
lung cancer 3
lying to patients 24

Macmillan Nurse 115, 118
Maguire, P. 21
Marie Curie nurse 118
Mental Health Act 109
metachlopromide 81
methadone 68, 103
metoclopramide 68, 80, 96, 97
midazolam 95, 96, 97
Mills, M. 63, 71
Misuse of Drugs Regulations (1985) 103
morphine 7, 63, 75–6, 89, 90, 95, 99, 103
motor neurone disease 9, 11–12, 68
Motor Neurone Disease Association 12, 49
Motor Neurone Disease nurses 12
multiple sclerosis 53, 58–9

Munk, W. 7, 75
muscarinic cholinergic 81

naproxen 89
nasogastric tubes 59
nausea 63, 64, 67, 68, 80
nervous tissue 77
Netherlands 50
neuralgia 78
neurological problems 8
neuropathic pain 77–9
non-opioid analgesics 72, 74
non-steroidal anti-inflammatory drugs
  (NSAIDS) 72
nurses see Macmillan; Marie Curie; Motor
  Neurone Disease; specialist
nursing service 118–19
nutrition 51, 59

octreotide 80
ondansetron 81
opioids 7, 67, 68, 74, 75, 78, 96, 99
  and dose calculation 95
  see also weak; strong
oropharyngeal local anesthetic 68
outcome improvement 64–5
outpatient clinics 117

pain 18, 63, 64
  abdominal 67
  management 71–9
    morphine 75–6
    neuropathic pain and adjuvant analgesics
      77–9
    strong opioid analgesics 75
    strong opioids 76–7
    weak opioid analgesics 74–5
    World Health Organization analgesic
      ladder 72–4
  total 35, 67
paracetamol 72, 74
Parkes, C. M. 8
Parkinson's disease 47, 58
patients and financial benefits 106–7
patient's outlook 15–20
  attention to detail 18–19
  problem list 19–20
  talking and listening 16–18
pentazocine 103

persistent vegetative state 49
personal experience 39–40
pethidine 103
Petrone, M. 6, 10
phenazocine 103
phenytoin 89
pholcodeine 68
physical symptom control 63–85
  advanced disease 64
  anticipation 65–6
  attention to detail 70
  constipation and diarrhoea 83
  continuity 70–1
  dyspnoea and cough 82
  evaluation and assessment 66–8
  explanation and information 68
  individualized treatment 68–9
  intractable vomiting 81
  last days of life 84–5
  nausea and vomiting 80
  outcome improvement 64–5
  pain management 71–9
  re-evaluation and supervision 69–70
physiotherapy 68
pioneers of palliative care 7–8
place 39
  of choice for dying 55–7
pneumonia 68
Porter, R. 45
post-herpetic neuralgia 78
prescribing controlled drugs 103–6
prioritization 38
private insurance 107
problem list 19–20
prochlorperazine 81, 89
professional attitudes 39
prognosis 24
psychological distress 67
psychosocial aspects 18, 29–41
  Balint, M. 36
  barriers 38–41
  burnout avoidance 40–1
  communication 37–8
  contexts of awareness 35–6
  dying, stages of 34–5
  improvements 30–1
  needs 31–3
  total pain 35

Rapid Response Teams 116
real-world history taking 25
rectally administered drugs 89
re-evaluation 69–70
regulations and statutory duties 103–12
  cremation form 109–12

death certification 107–9
death verification 107
drug use, unlicensed 106
financial benefits for patients 106–7
prescribing controlled drugs 103–6
renal cell carcinoma 31
respiratory problems 8, 9, 64
Respite at Home Teams 116
resuscitation 59
Royal College of Physicians 7

sadness 31, 32
St Christopher's Hospice 7
Saunders, C. 7–8, 35
scientific theory 33–6
sedation/sedatives 67, 89, 96
senna 75
sensitivity 22
serotonin 81
serum calcium 67
side-effects 78
  prevention 75, 76
sleep disturbances 64
social distress 67
specialist palliative care nurse 118–19
specialist palliative care services 115–19
spinal metastases 66
spiritual distress 67
state aid 106–7
statutory duties see regulations and statutory
    duties
steroids 79, 80, 96
stroke 8
strong opioid analgesics 75
strong opioids 76–7, 106
subcutaneous administration 89, 93, 97, 99
suicide 40
supervision 69–70
suppositories 67, 80
syringe driver 89–99
  attachment of loaded syringe 93
  boost button 94–5
  drug combinations 95
  drug dose changes 95–8
  drugs administered 95
  Graseby MS 16 and MS 26 90–1
  infusion care 98
  infusion commencement 93
  infusion preparation 92
  infusion rate 94
  infusion and time to take effect 94
  infusion-site irritation 98
  opioids and dose calculation 95
  preparation 92–3
  setting up 91–2

talking 16–18
teamwork 38–9
temazepam overdose 3
Terence Higgins Trust 49
Timmermans, S. 35
tiredness 39
total pain 35, 67
train of thought 32
trauma 77
tregeminal neuralgia 78
tricyclic antidepressants 79

uncontrolled symptoms 50
United Kingdom 71

United States 71
urinary retention 67

ventilation 59
vomiting 64, 80, 89, 90
  intractable 81

weak opioid analgesics 74–5
Williams, C. J. B. 3
work ethic 39
workload 38
World Health Organization 4
  analgesic ladder 72–4, 77